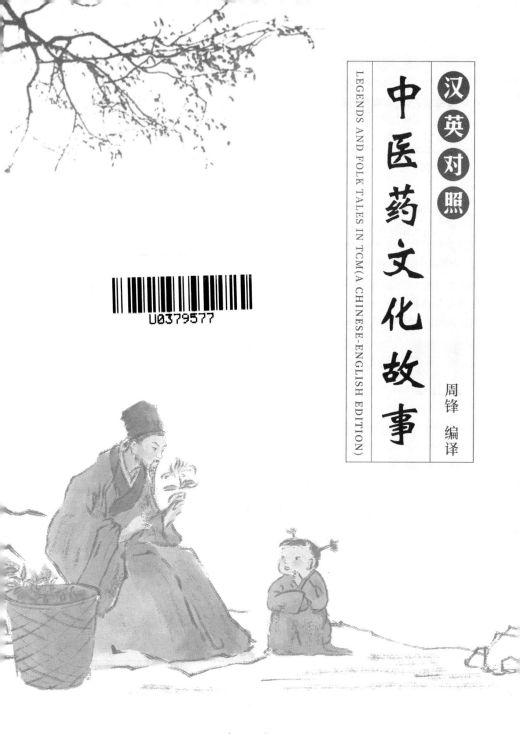

汉英对照

中医药文化故事

LEGENDS AND FOLK TALES IN TCM(A CHINESE-ENGLISH EDITION)

周锋 编译

U0379577

重庆大学出版社

内容提要

中医学是中华民族优秀传统文化的一部分，从中可以洞见中国的道学文化、儒学文化和佛学文化，对其进行传承和发扬具有重要的意义。同时，越来越多的外国友人对中医学产生了浓厚的兴趣。《中医药文化故事（汉英对照）》在此背景下应运而生，该书共三大部分，主题涵盖较为宽泛，主要涉及中医药重要著作和古中医学名家，重要中草药，以及与中医药相关的成语和俗语。该教材特色鲜明，所选用的小故事趣味性强，尤其适用于初学者和外国留学生的中医药教学，是一本能满足相应学习需求的汉英对照版教材。

图书在版编目（CIP）数据

中医药文化故事：汉英对照/周锋编译. -- 重庆：
重庆大学出版社，2019.10
ISBN 978-7-5689-1694-3

Ⅰ.①中⋯　Ⅱ.①周⋯　Ⅲ.①中国医药学—文化—汉、英　Ⅳ.①R2-05

中国版本图书馆 CIP 数据核字（2019）第 153117 号

中医药文化故事（汉英对照）

ZHONGYIYAO WENHUA GUSHI(HAN-YING DUIZHAO)

周　锋　编译
责任编辑：张晓琴　　版式设计：张晓琴
责任校对：刘志刚　　责任印制：赵　晟

*

重庆大学出版社出版发行
出版人：饶帮华
社址：重庆市沙坪坝区大学城西路 21 号
邮编：401331
电话：（023）88617190　88617185（中小学）
传真：（023）88617186　88617166
网址：http://www.cqup.com.cn
邮箱：fxk@ cqup.com.cn（营销中心）
全国新华书店经销
重庆升光电力印务有限公司印刷

*

开本：890mm×1240mm　1/32　印张：5　字数：193 千
2019 年 12 月第 1 版　　2019 年 12 月第 1 次印刷
ISBN 978-7-5689-1694-3　　定价：25.00 元

前　言

　　中医学是中华民族传统文化的一部分,具有浓厚的中国传统文化色彩,融入了中国的道学文化、儒学文化和佛学文化。而中医典籍的语言又是典型的古汉语的文学语言与哲学语言。五千多年来,中医药对中华民族的生存和繁衍、防病治病、强身健体,发挥了重大的作用。

　　中医药有自己一套独特的理论与体系。它强调人与自然是一个有机的整体,许多疾病是由于环境造成的;人体的各部分又是一个有机的整体,一个器官有病,必然影响到全身。

　　中医的理论主要是探索生命循环的本质和疾病产生的原因。它的阴阳、五行、气、血、津液、脏腑、经络等理论,充满辩证法,解释疾病产生的原因以及如何诊断、治病防病、强身健体等。

　　中医的诊断方法(望、闻、问、切)和诊疗方法(针灸、艾灸、拔罐、推拿、刮痧、食疗、中草药等)都是建立在它的生命理论和治疗体系上的。

　　中国古代名医华佗,发现阳春三月的青蒿的嫩叶,可治黄疸病;当代中医专家屠呦呦和她的研究团队,在研究了众多中医典籍和数千验方之后,发明了青蒿素,专治恶性疟原虫疟疾,从而挽救了数百万非洲人民的生命,获 2015 年诺贝尔医学与生物学奖。

　　每一年,都有大批的外国留学生来到中国的中医院校学习中医药。要掌握深奥的中医理论、精密的诊断方法和各种治疗方法,这对他们来说,是十分困难的事情,非下三五年的苦功夫不可。而编写《中医药文化故事(汉英对照)》一书,既可以夯实他们的中医药文化底蕴,又可以提高他们学习中医药的兴趣,这是我们编写此书的初衷。同时,这本书对于"中国传统文化走出去"和"讲好中国故事",是一次有益的尝试。

　　我们在中医药院校从事教学工作多年,得益于良好中国文化氛围的熏陶,且通过教习"医学英语"等课程,对中医的基本理论和文化底蕴有了一定的了解。同时,通过承担多批外国留学生的医学英语教学和课堂翻译工作,让我了解到中医翻译的不易。在伟大的中医药宝库面前,我们"什么也不是",就像一个旅者,远眺一个城市的夜景,只见一片灯光,心中充满了渴望与梦想。

在本书编译的过程中,得到了广西大学外国语学院、广西外国语学院原院长周仪教授的悉心帮助与指导,他扎实的语言知识底蕴、对中国传统文化的广泛涉猎以及严谨认真的治学态度,都是促使我们认真编译此书,使之尽快与读者见面的强大动力,在此向周仪教授和给予本书帮助的各位老师表示真诚感谢。

本书实为投石问路之举,限于本人水平浅陋,谬误在所难免,不当之处,万望专家与读者批评、指正。

编译者

2019 年 2 月

广西中医药大学

目　录

第一部分　中医名家与经典
Part One　TCM Celebrities and Classics

中医理论 ……………………………………………… 2

TCM Theory ……………………………………… 2

中医对病的认识 …………………………………… 3

The Chinese Attitude Towards Disease ………… 3

中医的图腾——葫芦 ……………………………… 4

Gourd—Totem of Chinese Medicine …………… 4

《黄帝内经》 ………………………………………… 7

The Yellow Emperor's Canon of Internal Medicine(Huang Di Nei Jing) …

…………………………………………………… 7

《本草纲目》 ………………………………………… 9

Compendium of Materia Medica ………………… 9

神农尝百草 ………………………………………… 11

Shennong Tasted Herbs ………………………… 11

扁鹊与牛黄 ………………………………………… 13

Bian Que and Niu Huang(Bezoar) …………… 13

扁鹊见秦武王 ……………………………………… 15

Bian Que Met King Wu of Qin ………………… 15

医圣张仲景 ………………………………………… 16

Zhang Zhongjing—The Sage of Traditional Chinese Medicine ……… 16

仲景诊病 …………………………………………… 18

A Story of Zhang Zhongjing …………………… 18

韩康卖药 …………………………………………… 19

Han Kang Sold Herbs …………………………… 19

神医华佗与乌鸡白凤丸 ·· 21

  The Great Doctor Hua Tuo and Wuji Baifeng Pills ············· 22

华佗与五禽戏 ·· 25

  Hua Tuo and Five Animals Play ······························ 25

曹操杀华佗 ·· 27

  Cao Cao Killed Hua Tuo ···································· 28

葛洪炼丹 ·· 30

  Ge Hong and Alchemy ······································ 30

药王孙思邈 ·· 32

  Sun Simiao, King of Medicine ······························ 32

苏东坡美食养生方 ·· 34

  Su Dongpo's Food Therapy ·································· 34

范仲淹：不为良相，愿为良医 ······································ 36

  Fan Zhongyan：Be a Loyal Minister or a Good Doctor ········· 36

钱乙自治 ·· 38

  Qian Yi Healed Himself ···································· 38

李时珍 ·· 40

  Li Shizhen ·· 40

喻嘉言救母子二人性命 ·· 42

  Yu Jiayan Saved Lives of the Mother and the Kid ············· 42

叶天士治红眼病 ·· 44

  Ye Tianshi's Treatment for Pinkeyes ························ 44

第二部分　中草药的故事

Part Two　Stories of Chinese Materia Medica

中草药 ·· 48

  Chinese Herbal Medicine ···································· 48

三七的故事 ································ 49

  The Story of Sanqi（Notoginseng Radix et Rhizoma）············ 49

仙鹤草 ··································· 51

  Crane Herb（Agrimoniae Herba）·················· 51

红景天 ··································· 53

  Hong Jing Tian（Rhodiolae Crenulatae Radix et Rhizoma）········ 53

益母草 ··································· 54

  Yi Mu Herb（Leonuri Herba）··················· 54

黄连 ···································· 56

  Huang Lian（Coptidis Rhizoma）·················· 57

断肠草（钩吻）····························· 59

  Intestines-broken Herb（Geldrmium Elegans）············ 59

夏枯草 ··································· 61

  The Story of Xiaku Grass（Prunellae Spica）············ 61

鱼腥草 ··································· 63

  Yu Xing Cao（Houttuyniae Herba）················ 63

金银花 ··································· 64

  Jin Yin Flower（Lonicerae Japonicae Flos）············ 64

茵陈 ···································· 66

  Yin Chen（Artemisiae Scopariae Herba）·············· 66

吴茱萸 ··································· 68

  Wu Zhu Yu（Euodiae Fructus）·················· 69

辛夷 ···································· 71

  Xin Yi（Magnoliae Flos）····················· 72

鹅不食草 ································· 74

  Goose-Not-Eat Grass（Centipedae Herba）············· 74

薏苡明珠 ································· 76

  Yiyi（Coicis Semen）······················ 76

石菖蒲 ··································· 78

Shi Chang Pu (Acori Tatarinowii Rhizoma) ·················· 78

豆蔻年华 ··· 79

Budding Beauty (Amomi Fructus Rotundus) ·············· 79

徐长卿 ··· 81

Xu Changqing (Cynanchi Paniculati Radix et Rhizoma) ·············· 81

人参 ··· 83

Ginseng (Ginseng Radix et Rhizoma) ························· 83

小和尚和人参的故事 ··· 85

The Story of a Little Monk and Ginseng ·················· 85

丹参 ··· 87

Dan Shen (Salviae Miltiorrhizae Radix et Rhizoma) ·············· 87

当归 ··· 89

Dang Gui (Angelica Sinensis Radix) ·························· 89

麝香 ··· 90

She Xiang (Moschus) ·· 90

山药 ··· 92

Shan Yao (Dioscoreae Rhizoma) ································· 92

枸杞子 ··· 94

Goji (Lycii Fructus) ·· 94

八珍汤 ··· 96

Ba Zhen Soup ··· 96

熟地治瘟疫 ··· 98

Shudi (Rehmanniae Radix Praeparata) Treated Plague ·············· 98

黄精 ··· 99

Huang Jing (Polygonati Rhizoma) ······························ 99

何首乌 ··· 100

He Shouwu (Polygoni Multiflori Radix) ···················· 100

橘井泉香 ··· 102

Well Water and Tangerine Leaves ····························· 102

葛根的传说 ·················· 103

The Legend of Gegen（Puerariae Lobatae Radix）·············· 103

麻沸散的发明 ················· 105

The Invention of Anesthesia Powder ············· 105

第三部分　成语与俗语
Part Three　Idioms and Proverbs

不可救药 ··················· 108

Beyond Remedy ················ 108

折肱 ····················· 109

Zhe Gong（Humerus）············· 109

病入膏肓 ··················· 110

Sick to the Vitals ·············· 110

大葫芦 ···················· 112

The Big Gourd ················ 113

讳疾忌医 ··················· 115

Refuse to Be Treated for Fear That Others Will Know About the Illness ···

················· 115

起死回生 ··················· 117

Make the Dead Come back to Life ·········· 118

洞见症结 ··················· 120

Sees Through the Crux ············· 120

妙手回春 ··················· 122

Bring a Patient Back to Health ··········· 122

天人相应 ··················· 124

Correspondence Between Human and the Nature ········· 124

悬壶济世 ··················· 126

Xuan Hu Ji Shi（To Practise Medicine to Save People）·············· 126

防微杜渐 ················ 127

    Be Precautious Before Hand ················ 127

贵人难医 ················ 129

    A Man Is Too Noble To Cure ················ 129

对症下药 ················ 131

    Suit the Medicine to the Illness ················ 131

刮骨疗毒 ················ 133

    Scrape Poison off the Bone ················ 133

杏林春暖 ················ 134

    Xing Lin Chun Nuan ················ 134

以毒攻毒 ················ 136

    Fight Poison with Poison ················ 137

杯弓蛇影 ················ 139

    Mistake the Shadow of a Bow in One's Cup As a Snake ·········· 139

骗子卖药 ················ 141

    A Swindler Sold Herbs ················ 141

怡悦疗法 ················ 142

    Pleasure Therapy ················ 142

激怒疗法 ················ 143

    Anger Therapy ················ 143

逗笑疗法 ················ 145

    Fun Therapy ················ 145

羞耻疗法 ················ 147

    Shame Therapy ················ 147

参考文献 ················ 149

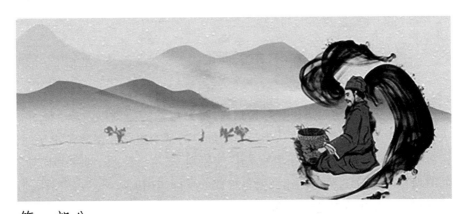

第一部分
Part One

中医名家与经典
TCM Celebrities and Classics

中医理论

中国传统医学是以阴/阳为基础的,与大自然的原则以及金、木、水、火、土五行互补,这些被古人认为是物理世界的基本组件。在遵守处方,中医(中国传统医学)的医生采取"治国"的原则,采用"君,臣,助手和向导"的原理,指的是通过处方的组成使各种部分发挥作用的战略。古中医医生由此把伦理和政治引进医学领域。

TCM Theory

Traditional Chinese medicine is based on *yin/yang*, with the opposing, complementary principles of nature and the five elements of metal, wood, water, fire and earth. These are believed by ancient Chinese to be the basic components of the universe. In complying prescriptions, traditional Chinese medicine doctors adopt the strategy of "governing a country"—the principle being to employ "monarch, minister, assistant and guide", which refers to the various roles played by the components of a prescription. Ancient TCM doctors thus introduced ethics and politics into the realm of medicine.

中医对病的认识

　　据中国宇宙观,一切生命都是起源于阴阳的结合。两者之间的和谐产生良好的健康;不和谐导致疾病。一个传统的中国药学理论假设是:病是由于阴阳的内部失衡产生的,所以治病的策略是恢复和谐,中国传统的医生用针灸、草药和特殊食品来帮助纠正阴阳的不平衡,直到身体恢复到健康状态。另一假设是,各器官有精神或物理功能,并且身体的所有部分都是紧密相连的。

The Chinese Attitude Towards Disease

　　According to the Chinese cosmology, all lives are born from the integration of *yin* and *yang*. Harmony between the two produces good health while disharmony leads to disease. One of the major assumptions of traditional Chinese medicine is that disease is due to an internal imbalance between *yin* and *yang*, and so the strategy is to restore harmony. Traditional Chinese doctors use acupuncture, herbs and special food to help correct *yin-yang* imbalance until the body returns to a healthy state. Another assumption is that each organ has a mental as well as a physical function, and all parts of the body are intimately connected.

中医的图腾——葫芦

葫芦既为食物、蔬菜，又可作器皿瓢饮。葫芦干后可以倒出很多种子，用以繁殖，与生殖崇拜有关。在广西瑶族的传统中，葫芦还与洪水时救了伏羲、女娲两兄妹的命有关。因此，葫芦是南方许多民族的图腾标志。

《后汉书》及葛洪的《神仙传》中记载：壶公，不知其姓名。费长房为市掾，忽见公从远方来，入肆卖药，人莫识之。卖药口不二价，治病皆愈。常悬一空壶于屋上，日入之后，公跳入壶中，人莫能见。唯长房楼上见之，知非常人也。长房乃自扫公座前地及供馔物，公受而不辞。如此积久，公知长房笃信，谓房曰："至暮无人时更来。"长房如其言往，公语房曰："见我跳入壶中时，即便效我跳。"长房依言，果不觉已入。唯见玉堂俨丽，楼台重门阁道，公左右侍者数十人。乃与长房共饮，酒器如拳许大，饮之至暮不竭。后长房求道，随从入山，能医疗众病，鞭笞百鬼。后失其符，为众鬼所杀。其治病皆能愈，并每语人曰：服此药必吐某物，某日当愈，言无不效。如所周知，历来卖药的常置药于壶中；炼丹术士更是置金丹于壶中。药铺市招，常以葫芦为标识鬻卖。因此葫芦为药肆、郎中标识无疑。俗话说"不知他葫芦里卖的什么药"。从上述故事可窥见葫芦在原始意识中与医药有不解之缘，本为互渗而来的图腾标记。

Gourd—Totem of Chinese Medicine

Gourd could be used as food, vegetable and ladle or utensil for drinking. The worship of reproduction is associated with gourd because gourd produces numerous seeds when dried. Among the traditions of the Yao nationality of Guangxi in China, gourd played a part in saving the lives of Fuxi and Nuwa, brother and sister, ancestors of the Chinese people, in the great flood. In fact, gourd has been a totem for many southern nationalities in China.

Both *Hou Han Shu* and Ge Hong's *Shen Xian Zhuan* described the following story. Hu, a senior, came from afar, nobody knew his name. Fei Zhangfang, a market administrator, saw him enter a shop to sell his medicines. Although the prices were non-negotiable, the medicines worked. The man often hung an empty gourd on the beam in his room and jumped into it after sunset each day. Zhangfang happened to see this from an upper floor, and began to understand that this man was not a common folk. He swept the floor of his room and presented Hu with food and drinks. The old man took all without hesitation. Each day, Zhangfang did the same. After a period of time, the old man was assured of Zhangfang's trust and told him, "Come at dusk when nobody's around." Zhangfang went as he had been told. Then the man said, "When I jump into the gourd, follow me immediately." Zhangfang followed him and was in the gourd before he knew it. Before him was a grand jade hall with numerous buildings and towers around, and intertwining doors and corridors. More than ten servants were waiting on Senior Hu. Then Zhangfang and Senior Hu enjoyed a feast. The drinking cup was as big as a man's fist and would never run dry till deep into the night. Later Zhangfang asked the man to teach him Taoism and followed him deep into the mountains. As a result, Zhangfang learned to heal diseases and even could lash out at ghosts. However, eventually he was killed by ghosts, after his magic talisman went missing. Whatever disease it was, Zhangfang could cure it. Each time he would tell the patient that the medicine would make him vomit something up and then the disease would be healed on a certain day. His words always came true. It is well-known to the Chinese people that a medicine seller by tradition puts his medicine in a gourd; and a Taoism alchemist hides his magic pills in a gourd at all times. Outside herbal shops, gourds are hung as a sign that there are medicines for sale. Therefore, if you see a gourd, you know that a herbal medicine shop or physician is around. Just as a

Chinese idiom goes "you don't know what kind of medicine he is selling in his gourd." All these stories indicate that gourds are intertwined with medicine in primitive thinking and function as the totem of Chinese medicine.

《黄帝内经》

　　《黄帝内经》，作者不详，是中国现存最早的一部医学经典。它包括《素问》与《针经》(又名《灵枢》)各9卷，共计18卷，162篇，但是部分章节年久失传。

　　《素问》以黄帝和天师岐伯问答的形式，着重阐述关于人体生理、病理等基本理论，《灵枢》则叙述针灸、经络、卫生保健等方面的问题。

　　《黄帝内经》初步建立了我国中医学的理论体系，一直指导着中医的临床实践，在我国医学史上占有重要的地位。《黄帝内经》已经引起国内外医学家和科学史家的重视，部分内容已相继翻译成日、英、德、法等国文字，日本等国家还出现了不少研究《黄帝内经》的著作。

The Yellow Emperor's Canon of Internal Medicine(Huang Di Nei Jing)

　　The Yellow Emperor's Canon of Internal Medicine, whose author is unknown, is the earliest medical classic in China. It includes two parts: *Plain Questions* and *Acupuncture Classic* (or *Miraculous Pivot*), and each of them comprises 9 volumes. The 18 volumes originally consist of 162 articles, but some of the chapters have been lost with the lapse of time.

　　In a question-and-answer form, *Plain Questions* recounts the discussion between the Yellow Emperor and his royal physician Qi Bo. It mainly sets forth the basic theories of physiology and pathology of the human body. *Miraculours Pivot* dwells upon acupuncture and moxibustion, main and collateral channels as well as hygiene and health care.

　　The Yellow Emperor's Canon of Internal Medicine lays the foundation for the theoretical systems of the traditional Chinese medicine, which has long guided the clinical practice of Chinese medicine and plays an important role in China's medical history. Its significance has caught the attention of medical scientists and historians of science both at home and abroad. Parts of the book have been translated into Japanese, English, German and French. Many treatises on *The Yellow Emperor's Canon of Internal Medicine* have been published in Japan, as well as in other countries.

《本草纲目》

《本草纲目》是一部药物学的洋洋巨著,也可以说是生物学上一部较早的百科全书。它不仅是祖国医学发展史上的光辉成就,也为世界医药学和生物学做出了重大的贡献。

《本草纲目》这部书在明代万历年间出版以后,很快就流传到了日本、朝鲜和越南。十七、十八世纪传入欧洲,立即得到各国的重视。先后被翻译成英文、法文、德文、俄文和拉丁文出版。英国生物学家达尔文在撰写关于进化论的著作(《人类的由来》)时,还引用了《本草纲目》中关于金鱼颜色的形成的史料,来说明动物的人工选择,可见这部著作的价值和影响是多么大。

这部巨著的作者是生活在明代嘉靖、万历年间的李时珍。李时珍最伟大的贡献是对"本草"的研究和整理方面。《本草》是专讲药物的,李时珍在长期的医疗实践中,发现以前的本草不仅缺漏较多,而且有不少错误,李时珍深知这些药书上的混乱和错误,会带来治疗上的严重后果,因此,他决心重新编写一部本草。《本草纲目》是李时珍倾注了毕生精力的不朽巨作。可惜,这部书定稿之后不久,他便与世长辞了,生前没有看到这部书的出版。

Compendium of Materia Medica

Compendium of Materia Medica is a monumental work of pharmacology, also known as an earlier encyclopedia in the field of biology. It acts not only as a brilliant achievement in TCM development, but also a momentous contribution to the world's medicine and biology.

Published in Wanli period of Ming Dynasty (1573-1620), the book spread rapidly to Japan, Korea, Vietnam, and then to Europe in the 17th and 18th centuries. It lured a worldwide attention and was highly valued by the world. It has also been translated and published in English, French, German, Russian and Latin. In his *In Human Variation And Origins*: *An Introduction To Biology And Evolution*, the British biologist Charles Robert Darwin (1809-1882) once consulted the book for historical data on the formation of skin colors of gold fish to demonstrate the artificial selection process of animals, a vivid evidence of the great value and influence of the book.

The author of this masterpiece is Li Shizhen. He was a great physician and pharmacologist in the Jiajing period and Wanli period of Ming Dynasty. His most significant contribution falls on the study and organizing of "herbal medicines", which was finally compiled into a monograph on medication. In his age-long medical practice, Li Shizhen found that there had been a great amount of mismatches and deficiencies and even some inaccuracies in the previous herbal medicine books, which, Li Shizhen affirmed, might lead to dangerous consequences. Given this fact, he was determined to write a book on herbal medicine. Li Shizhen dedicated all his lifetime to this immortal work. It was a pity that he passed away no sooner than the manuscript had just been finalized. He failed to witness the publication of the book in his life time.

神农尝百草

饮茶是中国文化的一个组成部分。

据陆羽《茶经》所载,中国饮茶最早要追溯到周朝(公元前1046—公元前222年):"茶之为饮,发乎神农氏,闻于鲁周公。"茶在中国已有四千年的历史了。相传有位传奇英雄叫神农,品尝了成百上千种植物,并分辨出哪些是有毒的,哪些是可以食用的,以此来防止人们吃到有毒的植物。据说他曾经一天中毒72次,后因咀嚼了一种开着白色花朵的长青树嫩叶而脱险了。神农的肚子是水晶般透明的。人们可以看见食物是如何通过胃和肠消化的。当他们看到这种嫩叶汁在他胃里上下洗涤,好似在检查什么,就称这种绿叶为"查",即寻找的意思。后来转命名为"茶",与"查"同音。

中国人民世世代代传颂这个故事,是为了表示崇敬和纪念这位中国农业和医学事业的开创者的功绩。

Shennong Tasted Herbs

Tea-drinking is a constituent part of Chinese culture.

According to Lu Yu's *Tea Classics*, tea-drinking in China can be traced back to the Zhou Dynasty (1046 B. C. – 222 B. C.), "Tea was discovered by Shennong and became popular as a drink in the State of Lu (1043 B. C. – 249 B. C.) because of Zhou Gong." Tea drinking in China has a history of four thousand years. As the legend has it, Shennong, a legendary hero, tasted hundreds of wild plants to see which were poisonous and which were edible, so as to prevent people from eating the poisonous plants. It is said that he was poisoned seventy-two times in one day and was saved by chewing some tender leaves of an evergreen plant with white flowers blossoming. Since he had a transparent belly, people could see how the food moved throughout his stomach and intestines. When they saw the juice of the tender leaves go up and down in the stomach as if it were searching for something, they called it "查(cha)" (meaning "search"). Later it was renamed "茶"(cha) having the same pronunciation of "查".

People told and retold this story from generation to generation, paying great respect to this ancestor, who pioneered agriculture and Chinese medicine.

扁鹊与牛黄

　　牛黄,是一味名贵的中药。相传,牛黄是我国古代医学家扁鹊在无意中发现的。一天,扁鹊正在桌上整理煅制好的金礞石。此时,邻居阳宝杀了一头病牛,发现牛胆囊中有些像石头样的东西,不知是何物,于是提着胆囊来向扁鹊请教。扁鹊剖开胆囊取出两枚"石头"放在桌上、仔细地琢磨。

　　回家不久的阳宝又惊叫着跑来说其父亲一口气上不来,在炕上抽搐不停。扁鹊急忙去阳宝家,只见阳宝的老父亲双眼上翻,喉中噜噜有声。扁鹊看罢,立即吩咐阳宝快到桌上把金礞石拿来研成末,给阳宝父亲灌下。须臾,阳宝的父亲就止住抽搐,气息也平静了。扁鹊回家时却发现桌上的两枚牛"石头"不见了。细寻之下,原来阳宝在慌乱中错把牛黄当金礞石拿去了。扁鹊思忖:"难道这种石头真的有豁痰定惊的功效?"

　　遂于次日,有意用其配药,给阳宝的父亲送去服之。不日,病奇迹般的好了。扁鹊就将这种黄牛胆内的深黄色之物命名为"牛黄"。

Bian Que and Niu Huang(Bezoar)

　　Niu Huang(Bezoar) is a blindly expensive traditional Chinese medicine. As the legend has it, it was accidently discovered by Bian Que, an ancient Chinese medical scientist. One day, Bian Que was sorting out the gold chloriti which had been calcined on the table. At that time, his neighbor Yang Bao killed a sick cow and found something like stone in the gallbladder. He didn't know what it was. So Yang Bao took the gallbladder to ask Bian Que. Bian Que opened the gallbladder and took out two "stones" on the table, watching them carefully.

　　After returning home for a while, Yang Bao hurriedly ran back and told

Bian Que that his father could not breathe and kept twitching on the bed. Bian Que hurried to Yang Bao's home and saw that the old man turned up his eyes, making noise in his throat. Bian Que asked Yang Bao to bring the chloriti quickly which were put on the table in his home. He grounded it into powder and poured it down the throat of the patient. After a while, Yang Bao's father stopped twitching and subsequently his breath was going calm. When Bian Que returned home, he found the two cow "stones" on the table missing. Under careful examinations, he found that Yang Bao mistook it for the gold chloriti. Bian Que thought: Does the "stone" have the effect of clearing away phlegm and calming the frigntening?

The next day, he used it as a component to make medicine and sent it to Yang Bao's father. Within a few days, the old man was miraculously fully recovered. Bian Que named the dark-yellow stone in the sick cow's gallbladder as Niu Huang.

扁鹊见秦武王

扁鹊是古时候有名的神医。一天,当秦武王把自己的病情告诉扁鹊,扁鹊准备予以治疗。

秦武王的近臣说:"大王的病在耳朵和眼睛之间,这是很难治的。如果处理不当,就可能把耳朵搞聋,把眼睛弄瞎。"秦武王听了近臣的话,犹豫是否让扁鹊治病。

扁鹊听了很生气,对武王说:"君王既然跟懂得医理的人商量治病,却又听信不懂医理的人胡言乱语,这怎么能治好您的病呢? 如果用这种办法来管理秦国的政事,秦国很快就会灭亡啊!"

Bian Que Met King Wu of Qin

Bian Que(407 B.C.-310 B.C.) was a famous doctor in ancient China. One day he was going to cure some disease for King Wu of Qin(329 B.C.-307 B.C.) after the King informed him of his illness.

But the King's favorite officials said, " Your Majesty's illness resides between the eye and the ear. It is hard to deal with. If it is not treated properly, your ears will get deaf and eyes blind. Hearing this, the King hesitated whether to let Bian Que treat the disease or not.

When Bian Que heard of this, he was very angry and said to the King, " Your Majesty wants the doctor to cure your disease, but listen to those who do not know medicine and treatment. How can you get your sickness cured? If you handle the state affairs like that, the country is sure to go to its doom."

医圣张仲景

与华佗一样,张仲景也是东汉时期的名医,尤其对伤寒病最有研究。

公元196—219年,战乱频繁,瘟疫大为流行,病死的人很多。张仲景的家族原有200多口人,不到10年的时间,就病死了2/3,其中70%的人是患伤寒这种流行病死的。那时候所说的伤寒病,是包括霍乱、痢疾、肺炎、流行性感冒等一些急性传染病。在东汉末年,大多数医生对这种流行病还束手无策,没有对症治疗的办法,所以成百上千的人被这种病夺去了生命。经过长期努力,张仲景总结出一整套关于伤寒病的病理、诊断及治疗、用药的理论和方法。他认为伤寒病从初起到病危,有一个逐步发展的过程,在不同的阶段,对不同的病人,应当有不同的治疗方法。张仲景一边行医,一边总结自己的临床经验,记录最行之有效的方剂。在多年行医经验的基础上,他撰写了一部《伤寒杂病论》,这部医书是中医的经典著作,历代医家都视为必读之书。

目前,各中医药大学都将此书作为必修的课程。张仲景以他自己的杰出贡献被后人尊称为"医圣"。

Zhang Zhongjing—The Sage of Traditional Chinese Medicine

Zhang Zhongjing, lived in the Eastern Han Dynasty (25 – 220), was a doctor as famous as Hua Tuo. He especially specialized in the typhoid fever.

From 196 to 219, warlords fought in chaos and plagues spread widely. Numerous people died of contagions. In Zhang Zhongjing's kindred, there had been over two hundred kinship members, but two thirds of them died of the disease within ten years. Among them, seventy percent died of the contagious typhoid. The so-called typhoid at that time included cholera, dysentery, pneumonia, flu and some other acute contagious diseases. In the late period of the Eastern Han Dynasty, most doctors felt helpless to these diseases, for there was no remedy right to cure them. As a result, thousands of people lost their lives. For that reason, Zhang Zhongjing researched the diseases for years and summed up a complete system of theories on pathologh, diagnosis, therapy and prescriptions for typhoid fevers. He maintained that the typhoid developed gradually from the initial attack till the crucial dying stage. Treatments should be varied according to different individuals at the different stages of the disease development. Zhang Zhongjing kept on summing up his clinic experience while he was practicing medicine, noting down those effective prescriptions. Based on his years' practice of medicine, he worked out a monograph, *Shang Han Za Bing Lun* (*Teatise on Febrile and Miscellanesous Diseases*). This is a classic work on traditional Chinese medicine. Doctors of all generations deemed it as a must-read book.

Now all the TCM universities in China assign it as a compulsory course. In memory of him, Zhang Zhongjing was admired as a medical sage in honor of his significant contribution to TCM.

仲景诊病

据史学著作记载,张仲景遇到侍中王仲宣时,当时仲宣只有二十多岁,仲景对他说:"你得了病,到了四十岁眉毛会脱落,眉毛脱光半年之后将会死亡。"并告诉他,服药五石汤才能治好这个病。王仲宣嫌张仲景的话逆耳不恭,接受了他的药方却不听从劝告服药。过了三天,张仲景又见到王仲宣,问他服药了没有,仲宣回答已经服过了。张仲景说:"从您的面色症候来看,根本不像服过五石汤的样子,您为什么这样轻视自己的生命呢?"王仲宣仍然避而不答。

二十年后,仲宣的眉毛果然脱落,眉落后一百八十七天便去世了,就像仲景预言的那样。

A Story of Zhang Zhongjing

According to historical records, when the Privy Counselor Wang Zhongxuan was only 20 years old, he met Zhang Zhongjing, who told him that, "You have got a disease. Your eyebrows will fall off when you're forty years old and in half a year you will die." He advised him to take Five Stone Decoction to cure the disease. Wang Zhongxuan felt it harsh to hear, so he just accepted the prescription without taking it. Three days later, Zhang Zhongjing met Wang Zhongxuan again and asked him whether he had taken the medicine, Zhongxuan lied that he had already taken the medicine. Zhang Zhongjing said, "Judging from the symptom of your complexion, you haven't taken the decoction. Why do you take your own life so lightly?" Wang Zhongxuan fought shy of answering.

Twenty years later, Zhongxuan's eyebrows really fell off and died after 187 days. Zhang Zhongjing's prediction was demonstrated.

韩康卖药

汉朝时期,出身豪门的韩康不愿入仕当官,经常游名山大川采药到长安市场上去卖,三十年如一日,坚持言不二价。一天,一个牙痛不止的老太婆前来买药。忍不住对韩康讨价还价,只见韩康摆了摆手,严肃认真地说:"做生意,靠的是'信用'。所以,我从未虚报价格占人家的便宜,也从不接受客人的砍价。我的药,全是货真价实的灵药,绝对童叟无欺!"老太婆见韩康口气这么坚决,知道再讲也砍不下价,就买了一个钱的牙痛药走了。

城里的居民经过仔细打听,才知道摆这个药摊的人,原来就是赫赫有名的韩康!于是,大家一有什么病就都到他这里来买药,而且,也没有人尝试与他讲价。

有一次,一个女子向韩康买药,讨价还价,女子说她早就知道韩康言不二价。韩康叹息自己隐名避世还是被人认出,就隐遁于霸陵山中。

Han Kang Sold Herbs

During the Han Dynasty (206 B. C. – 220 B. C.), Han Kang, a wealthy man, was reluctant to be a government officer. He visited the famous mountains to gather herbs and sold them in Chang'an market. Moreover, he refused to bargain for 30 years. One day, an old woman who had toothache came to buy the medicine and she wanted to get some discount from Han. "A good business deals on faith. Therefore, the price of my medicine is all the same. I will never accept any bargain. All my herbs are genuine." Han Kang said seriously. The old woman realized that she could not make a bargain, so she bought some and left.

Local residents finally found that the man who sold herbs on the market was

Han Kang. Therefore, everyone would like to buy medicine from him and no one tried to bargain with him.

One day, a woman wanted to buy some medicine from Han and tried to bargain with him. Of course, it was no use. Then she said she had already known that Han Kang's herbs had set price. Han Kang sighed that he concealed his identity in the market but finally was recognized by people. Then he went to live in seclusion in the Baling Mountains.

神医华佗与乌鸡白凤丸

说起乌鸡白凤丸的由来,可谓历史渊源久远,最早可以追溯到三国时期的华佗。

有一年,华佗在徐土(今徐州)游学行医。他的堂兄用小车把华佗母亲推来了。华佗见母亲年老病危,行动喘息,说话气短,四肢无力,心里十分焦急。华佗母亲拉着儿子的手,不禁泪流满面。华佗为了安慰母亲,便把他在外面苦求医学的经过说了一遍。他母亲听了十分高兴,说:"儿呀!只要你能学到治病本事,为贫苦人家治好病,为娘在九泉之下也就瞑目了。现在我已年老,又病成这个样子,想在临死之前再见你一面,就请你堂兄把我送来,咱娘儿俩说两句话,娘就安心了。"华佗一听,伤心地哭了起来,含着泪把母亲的病仔细诊察了一遍,见脉沉迟无力,生命危在旦夕,立即用人参煎汤给母亲喝,病情略有好转;但一停药,病又加重。华佗见此情形,说:"母亲,您抱病前来看望孩儿,孩儿未能尽孝,心中实在难过,先请堂兄送您回家,带点药路上吃,孩儿把几个病人安排一下,随后即回。"母亲有气无力地说:"我也知道自己不行了,如死在外面也会难为你;你快把病人安排安排,不要耽误了人家的病,这是做医生的道德。"

华佗把兄长叫到一旁悄悄嘱咐说:"兄长,母病危重,六脉欲绝,估计不出三天,将要去世,请你路上小心照顾;我已准备好人参汤和急救药,路上代茶饮,以防中途去世,我随后赶回。"华佗含泪送走母亲后,忙把尚未治愈的病人,一一安排妥当,第二天起早就回家了。走了一天一夜终于到家了,到家一看母亲不但没死,反而能坐起来说话。华佗惊喜交集,心中不由疑惑起来:这是怎么回事呀?难道我诊断有误?华佗随即问堂兄:"你在路上给母亲吃过什么呀?"堂兄想了一会说:"在回来的那天晚上,住在一个小庄上,婶娘想喝口鸡汤,全村九户人家,养的都是母鸡,都舍不得卖。只有一家喂了一只公鸡,商量了半天,才把这只公鸡买来,借了个锅,熬了些汤,我把带来的人参汤和急救药放在鸡汤里一煮,让她老人家喝了一碗,她感觉很舒服,半夜又喝了一碗,第二天早上,全温给老人家喝了。回到家,老人家感到病好多了。"

华佗又问:"你买的鸡是什么样的?"

"白毛、凤头、皮肉都是黑的。"

华佗听罢,心想:白毛、黑皮、黑肉,头上羽毛如凤,再加上人参汤,难道是它起的作用?立即记下,于是到街上买了一只白毛黑皮的凤头鸡,按原法煮给母亲喝。华佗母亲的病逐渐好转了。原来人参大补元气而补五脏,乌鸡滋养阴血而补肝肾,有气血同补,阴阳双调之功效。后来,华佗又用此法,治好了许多患有同样病症的人。

The Great Doctor Hua Tuo and Wuji Baifeng Pill

Speaking of origin of Wuji Baifeng Pill, it has a long history. The story can be dated back to the period of Three Kingdoms(184-280), and a doctor called Hua Tuo must be mentioned.

Once upon a time, Hua Tuo(145-208) was practising medicine in Xutu (now Xuzhou). His cousin wheeled his mother in a small cart to see him. Hua Tuo saw that his old and ill mother felt short of breath, with myasthenia of limbs. He was very worried. Hua Tuo's mother, holding her son's hands, burst into tears. In order to comfort his mother, Hua told her his experience in studying medicine. His mother was very pleased and said, "My son! As long as you can obtain the skill of treatment, and cure the disease for the poor, I will not feel regret when I die. Now that I am old and ill, I would like to see you again before dying, so I ask your cousin to send me here. Having chatted with you, I have no regrets." Hua Tuo can not help crying as he heard these words. With tears in his eyes, he examined his mother's disease carefully and found that her pulse was too weak and her life was in danger, so he decocted the medicinal ginseng for her immediately. His mother got better slightly. However, once she stopped drinking the medicine, the disease got worse. Hua Tuo saw the situation and said, "Mom, you came to see me, but I am sorry that I had to work, so I'll ask my cousin to send you home first. Some medicines are prepared for you on the way, and I will be back soon." His mother said, "I know I am dying. I don't mean to be hard on you. Don't delay the patient's treatment since you are a doctor."

Hua Tuo called his brother to walk aside and whispered to him, "Our mom is seriously ill, and her pulses were feeble. She may pass away in three days. Please take care of her. I have prepared ginseng soup and some first-aid medicine, which can replace the tea on the road. I will be back as quick as possible." With tears in his eyes, Hua Tuo sent his mother away and soon arranged the patients who had not been treated, and then he went home early the next morning. After a day and a night walking, he finally reached home. When he arrived, he saw his mother still alive! Even better! She could sit up and talk. Hua Tuo was so surprised and happy, but also confused: What happened? Did I diagnose her wrongly? Then he asked his cousin, "What did you give our mom to eat on the way home?" The cousin thought for a moment and said, "On the way home, we put up in a small village for a night. Mom wanted to have some chicken soup, but all the nine families in the village raised only hens to lay eggs and no one was willing to sell there. Only a family fed a cock. Upon persuading, the family finally agreed to sell it to us. I borrowed a pot and cooked some chicken soup with the ginseng and the first-aid medicine we had bought with us, and then let our mom drink. She felt very comfortable. At midnight she drank the soup again, and the next morning, she drank up all the soup. When we were back home, our mom felt much better."

Hua Tuo asked once more, "What kind of chicken did you buy?"

"The one with white hair, phoenix head and black flesh."

Hua Tuo committed it to memory: white chicken, black skin, black meat, head feather like phoenix, with some ginseng. Did the cock really play a role?

He wrote down the prescription and bought the same white chicken. According to his cousin's method, Hua Tuo cooked the soup for his mom. His mother's illness gradually recovered. The pharmacodynamics is that the ginseng has the function of tonifying primordial qi and the five internal organs, and the chicken can nourish yin-blood liver and kidney, having the function of tonifying qi and blood and taking care of both Yin and $Yang$. Later, Hua Tuo cured many people of the same symptoms with this prescription.

华佗与五禽戏

华佗非常重视体育锻炼对人体健康的作用。华佗说："人体必须经常劳动，但不能过度。经常活动能使消化能力增强，血脉畅通，不易发生疾病。正如门轴一样，天天转动，就不会长蛀虫。"华佗这个看法是合乎科学道理的。

华佗是古代医疗体育的创始人之一。他根据"流水不腐，户枢不蠹"的原理，创造了一种叫作"五禽之戏"的体育运动。这种体育运动就是摹仿虎、鹿、熊、猿、鸟五种禽兽运动姿态的体操。第一种动作是摹仿虎的前肢扑捉的姿态；第二种动作是摹仿鹿扬伸头颈的姿态；第三种动作是摹仿熊侧卧的姿态；第四种动作是摹仿猿的脚尖纵跳的姿态；第五种动作是摹仿鸟的双翅飞翔的姿态。摹仿这五种动物姿态，可以使周身关节、脊背、腰部、四肢都得到舒展，得到抻拔活动。体质衰弱的人，练了"五禽之戏"，可以使体魄健壮起来；患病的人，练了"五禽之戏"，可以加速康复的进程；年迈的人，练了"五禽之戏"，可以容颜焕发，精神旺盛。

华佗弟子吴普，由于几十年坚持做"五禽之戏"，活到九十多岁，仍然步履轻捷，耳聪目明，牙齿坚固。可见，"五禽之戏"是行之有效的健身法。

Hua Tuo and Five Animals Play

Hua Tuo attached great importance to the effect of physical exercise on human body. "The human body must work often, but not excessively," said Hua Tuo. "Regular activity makes the digestive system strong, the blood vessels smooth, and disease free. Like the door-axis, if it turns every day, it will not get worm-eaten." Hua Tuo's view is quite in line with scientific principles.

Hua Tuo was one of the founders of ancient medical sports. He created a sport named "Five Animals Play" based on the principle that "running water is never stale and a door-hinge never gets worm-eaten." This sports is a kind of gymnastics, which imitates the movements and postures of tiger, deer, bear, ape and bird. The first movement is to imitate the tiger's forelimb catching prey, the second, to copy the deer's raising of its head and neck, the third, the bear lying on the side, the fourth, to model oneself on the ape's toe-jumping, and the fifth, to simulate the wings of the flying birds. By imitating these five animals, one can make the body joints, back, waist and limbs get stretched. A weak man may become physically strong by practicing "Five Animals Play". Those who are ill can speed up the process of recovery by practicing the "Five Animals Play", too. The old man, who has practiced the "Five Animals Play", can be radiant and energetic.

Wu Pu, one of Hua Tuo's disciples, lived to nineties because he had been practising the "Five Animals Play" for several decades. He had smart ears, good eyesight and strong teeth, and he could still walk with light steps at his nineties. It can be seen that "Five Animals Play" is an effective way to fitness.

曹操杀华佗

历史上的华佗，是一代名医。他出生在汉末沛国谯县，也就是现在的安徽亳县，是东汉末期医学家。华佗一生行医各地，精通内科、外科、儿科、针灸各科，尤其擅长外科，因此在当时的中国很有声誉。特别是他发明的"麻沸散"，在世界上前所未有，成为当今医学界医生动手术为病人麻醉的麻醉药。当然，华佗发明的"五禽戏"，也是医学上重大的发明创造，是中国现代体育运动、气功运动，甚至是武术界健身运动的始祖。因此，华佗被后人称为外科圣手、外科鼻祖。

曹操患有头风病，每次复发都头痛欲裂，十分痛苦。听说沛国谯县（今安徽亳县）的华佗医术很有名，便把他召来，留在身边专为自己诊治。头风再发作时，华佗只要针刺"鬲腧"一个穴位，病就好了。华佗在京日子久了，十分思念家乡亲人，便对曹操说："刚刚接到家里来信，家中有事，我必须请假回家一趟。"曹操只好答应了他的请求。华佗在家乡为百姓治病，实在不愿意回去侍候权贵，便以妻子有病为由，几次捎信给曹操，要求延长假期。

曹操多次命下属写信要华佗回去，又下令让郡县地方官催他回京，他都借口妻子病未好拒绝上路。曹操十分恼怒，立刻派人前去查核，并说："如果他的妻子确实有病，赏赐四十斛小豆，放宽假期；如果他妻子没有病，马上拘捕进京。"那人抓住华佗，把他关在许昌的监狱里。曹操的一位参赞催促曹操："华佗的医术很好，与人的生死有关，还是把他放了！"曹操不听，立刻下令处决华佗。当华佗去世前，他拿出一本书，对狱吏说："这本书可以拯救生命。"当狱吏不接受它的时候，华佗就把书烧了。

后来，曹操的儿子蜀处于危急关头，他叹了口气说："我真后悔杀了华佗，不然孩子就不会死了。"

Cao Cao Killed Hua Tuo

Born in Pei County(now Boxian, Anhui Province), Hua Tuo is a famous doctor as well as a medical scientist in the late Eastern Han Dynasty(25-220). He practiced medicine in his life all around the country, and was most proficient in internal medicine, surgery, pediatrics, acupuncture and other subjects, especially in surgery. He was extremely celebrated in China at that time. In particular, what he invented named "powder for anesthesia" is unprecedented in the world, and it became the narcotic which has been used for the operation. Besides, the "Five Animals Play" he invented is also an important invention and the ancestor of China modern sport, Qigong and even martial arts. In short, he was known as the surgical originator.

Cao Cao suffered from Toufeng syndrome, and he had a splitting headache every time it recurred. He heard of Hua Tuo's fame and sent someone to summon Hua Tuo to his side to serve him only. Each time his bad headache happened again, Hua Tuo would use the acupuncture needle to stimulate the "Ge Shu" acupoint, and then the pain would fade away. Hua Tuo had been in the capital city for such a long time that he missed his home and family. He said to Cao Cao,"I got a letter from my family and I want to go home for a vacation, may I?" Thinking for a long time, Cao Cao finally agreed,"I am really not willing to agree but I have to as you need some rest." When Hua Tuo returned to his hometown, he treated the poor people who got sick. He did not want to go back to serve the king anymore, so he sent letters to Cao Cao several times with the excuse of his wife's illness and asked for more days off.

Cao Cao ordered his subordinates to write a letter to Hua Tuo and asked the county magistrate to urge him to go back to the capital city. Hua Tuo refused again and again with the excuse of his wife's illness. Therefore Cao was very angry and immediately sent a man to check it out, saying, "If his wife was ill, give 40 *hu* (9.6 kilograms) of red beans to Hua Tuo and extend the leave. If not, you must arrest him, and take him back to the Capital." The man seized Hua Tuo and sent him to prison in Xuchang. One counsellor of Cao Cao said to him, "Hua Tuo has exquisite medical skills, and he can save people's life, please set him free." Turning a deaf ear to him, Cao Cao sentenced Hua Tuo to death immediately. Before he died, Hua Tuo took out a book and said to the warder, "This book can save lives." But the warder dare not accept it. Then Hua Tuo burned the book.

Later, when Cao Cao's son Shu was seriously ill, he sighed and said, "I regret having killed Hua Tuo. Otherwise, my child would be saved."

葛洪炼丹

晋朝(265—420)是司马氏篡夺曹魏而建立的政权。在篡位过程中,司马氏一方面大肆屠杀曹魏王室,另一方面残酷镇压拥护曹魏的天下士人。因为在儒家思想中,曾作为曹魏臣子的司马氏伐魏自立,是大逆不道、不得人心的,司马氏只得以高压的手段打击士人,让他们不得过问政治。

在这种形势下,士人谈论现实会招致杀身之祸,于是转向自我,转向自身,老庄思想大行其道,追求长生不老,关注练功养生,服炼仙丹。炼丹就是把各种被认为益寿的物质掺和在一起,以火煮炼。古人以为经过长时间煮炼的物质有助于延年益寿,长期服食可长生不老。炼丹也就成了古代化学的开端。

西晋人葛洪是炼丹的著名人物。自幼家里贫困,但勤奋好学,先学儒术,后好神仙养生之术。著有《抱朴子》一书,除讲神仙外,对炼丹论述颇多。

据史书记载,葛洪的祖父学道得仙,被称为“葛仙公”。葛洪得祖上真传,精悉炼丹之法。做了一段时间的官之后,就以年老为借口,远离西晋国都建康(今南京),请求做交址(今越南北部)令。皇帝认为交址地处偏远,阻止他去。葛洪说:“我去交址并无其他的想法,只是那地方有丹而已。”皇帝终于允诺了,于是葛洪携家室南行,至交址罗浮山炼丹,活到八十一岁,在古代也算是高寿了。

后来,“葛洪炼丹”这一典故,用来指避世养生。

Ge Hong and Alchemy

Jin Dynasty(265-420) was a regime established by Sima clan who usurped Cao's power of Wei (220 - 265). In his usurping process, the Sima clan massacred Cao's royal family on the one hand, and on the other hand, ruthlessly suppressed Cao's supporters, the Confucianists. Once being confucianists and having served Cao, the Sima clan knew that it was an unfilial thing to usurp the power. So the Sima clan had to suppress the people ruthlessly so that they dared not interfere in politics.

Under this circumstance, people who dared to talk about social reality would be killed, conversations about reality would lead to the speakers' death. So scholars turned to think about their own interesting thing—Zhuangzi's philosophy to pursue eternal life. Training to keep fit and the pursuit of immortals became popular among the people. Quite a lot of people felt interested in alchemy, trying to make immortal pills, which is said to be a mixture of all kinds of things that could prolong one's life refined in a stove for a long time. The ancients thought that the material that had been refined for a long time would help to maintain one's youthful vigour. Alchemy was the beginning of ancient chemistry in China.

Ge Hong was a famous figure of alchemy in the Western Jin Dynasty (265 - 316). He was poor but diligent when young. He wrote the book *Bao Pu Zi*, which contains not only the way of being immortals but also a lot of statements about alchemy.

According to historical classics, Ge Hong's grandfather had learned the way to be immortal, known as "Ge Xian Gong" (meaning "the fairy old man"). Ge Hong had learned from his ancestors and was good at alchemy. After being a government official for a period of time, he quit his office on the excuse that he was too old to stay in Jiankang (now Nanjing), the capital city, and requested to be a magistrate at Jiaozhi (now Northern Vietnam). The emperor thought that the place was too far and prevented him from going there. "I have no other ideas to go there, except that there was *Dan* (elixir)", he said. The emperor finally promised, so Ge Hong went to the south with his family, and lived there to eighty-one years old, a long life in ancient times.

Later, the allusion of "Ge Hong's Alchemy" refers to keeping away from the civil world and enjoying a leisure life.

药王孙思邈

药王孙思邈,隋唐时人,有《千金方》传世。民间流传的关于他的神奇故事不胜枚举。

有一次,孙思邈行医途中,遇到四个人抬着一口薄棺材向郊外的荒丘走去,后面跟着哭得跟泪人似的老婆婆。孙思邈定睛细看,发现从棺材的底缝里滴出几滴鲜血,便赶紧上前挡棺询问详情。原来棺材里是老婆婆的独生女儿,因难产刚死不久,胎儿仍在孕妇的肚子里。孙思邈听罢寻思:这个产妇可能还有救。于是,请求抬棺材的人赶紧撬开棺盖。只见产妇面色蜡黄,伸手摸脉竟发现还有微弱的跳动。他赶紧取出随身携带的银针,选准穴位,扎了下去,并采用捻针手法,加大力度。过了一会儿,"死去"的产妇竟然奇迹般地睁开了双眼,苏醒过来,同时腹中的胎儿也生出来了,发出一声清脆的啼哭。老婆婆见孙思邈一针救了两条性命,倒头便拜,四个抬棺的也长跪不起。

从此,孙思邈能起死回生的声名传开了,被人称为"活神仙"。

Sun Simiao, King of Medicine

Sun Simiao, King of Chinese herbal medicine, lived at the period of Sui and Tang Dynasties. His work *Qianjin Fang* has been passed down from generation to generation. Countless amazing stories about him spread in the folklore.

Once, Sun Simiao was practicing medicine on a tour and met four people carrying a thin coffin and going to the outskirts of barren hills, followed by an old lady who was full of tears. Sun looked carefully and found a few drops of blood dripping from the bottom of the coffin. Therefore, he came forward quickly to inquire for details. It turned out that the only daughter of the old woman was lying in the coffin, who had just died of childbirth and the fetus was still in her belly. Sun thought she might still have a chance to be saved. Hence, he asked the carriers to open the coffin immediately. He saw the "dead" woman with a sallow face and a weak pulse. Sun took out the silver needle in no time and picked the acupoint accurately, stuck and twisted the needle to increase the effect. After a while, the "dead" puerpera opened her eyes miraculously and came to life. At the same time, the baby came out with a sound cry. When the old woman saw that he had saved two lives with one needle, she fell down on her knees to worship Sun and the four carriers also prostrated on the floor.

Since then, Sun Simiao's reputation of making the dead come back to life has spread far and near and he is known as a "living immortal".

苏东坡美食养生方

宋代大文学家苏东坡不仅精通中医药学,也是一位美食养生家。他经常会摸索出一些既能治病保健,又能满足美食的养生方。苏东坡经常到山野里去发掘一些药食两用山草野味。一次,他走到一片稻田附近,突然看见他平时喜爱吃的野荸(即现在所说的荸荠),便想解解馋,于是用衣服捧着荸荠来到附近的寺院,借用灶火煮粥。方法是将荸荠 500 克,大米 100 克,生姜适量,煮成荸羹。荸羹不仅可以补充维生素 C,还有清热、利尿、平肝、和血、化痰的作用。

苏东坡还爱吃玉糁羹(山芋煮成的)。他经常下厨自己煮着吃,并且称这是健脾益气的佳品。中医史书也记载,山芋是块茎类食物,富含蛋白质、钙、磷、铁、胡萝卜素、维生素 B 族、维生素 C 等。可益脾和胃,治淋巴结肿大。外用可以帮助消肿、镇痛。麦门冬饮也是苏东坡喜欢的饮品,他将麦门冬饮制成具有口腔保健、安神催眠的家常饮料。并作诗说:"一枕清风值万钱,无人肯卖北窗眠。开心暖胃门冬饮,知是东坡手自煎。"麦门冬是中药中补阴的上品,有益阴养胃、润肺清心的功能。用于咽干口渴、大便燥结,也可用于心烦失眠、心悸盗汗等症。它的具体做法是,一次取少量麦门冬,像泡茶叶一样沏水喝。每天喝一二杯即可。

Su Dongpo's Food Therapy

Su Dongpo, a great man of letters in the Song Dynasty, was a gourmet and good at traditional Chinese medicine as well. He always searched for some recipes which could not only treat some illnesses but also help people keep fit. He often went to the mountains to find some wild herbs for medicine and food. Once, he came to a rice field and saw his favorite food, the water chestnuts, by chance. So, he grabbed some and wrapped them with his clothes to the nearby temple and cooked them. He used 500g of water chestnuts, 100g of rice and some ginger to boil them into porridge. Full of vitamin C, water chestnut can clear heat, promote diuresis, calm liver, activate blood and resolve phlegm.

He was also fond of "Yu San Geng"(meaning "sweet potato porridge"). He always cooked it by himself and said that it was good for strengthening spleen and nourishing *qi*. According to the Chinese historical Medicine records, the sweet potato is a kind of tuber food and rich in protein, calcium, phosphorus, iron, carotene, vitamin B and vitamin C. It benefits the spleen and the stomach and cures lymph node enlargement. It can help to relieve swelling and ease pain. "Mai Men Dong Drinks"(meaning "a drink made from Mai Men Dong, a newish food") was one of Su Dongpo's favorite beverages. He made it a home drink which had functions of maintaining oral health, soothing effect and hypnotic action. He also wrote a poem: A pillow in the wind is worth thousands of coins, no one will give up sleeping by the north window. Happiness and warm stomach are guaranteed by Men Dong drinks, you should know it is made by Su Dongpo. Mai Men Dong is the top nourishing food, with functions of supplementing *yin*, nourishing the stomach, moistening the lung and clearing away the heart-fire. It is used to cease dry throat and thirst, dry feces, insomnia, heart palpitations as well as night sweats. The method to make it is simple: take a small amount of Mai Men Dong, put it into a glass, and then pour in the boiling water. The drink is done. Drinking one or two glasses a day will keep you fit.

范仲淹:不为良相,愿为良医

宋代名儒范仲淹,当他困顿的时候,有一次到祠堂求签,问以后能否当宰相,签词表明不可以。他又求了一签,祈祷说:"如果不能当宰相,愿意当良医",结果还是不行。于是他长叹说:"不能为百姓谋利造福,不是大丈夫一生该做的事。"

后来,有人问他:"大丈夫立志当宰相,是理所当然的,您为什么又祈愿当良医呢? 这是不是有一点太卑微了?"

范仲淹回答说:"有才学的大丈夫,固然期望能辅佐明君治理国家,造福天下,哪怕有一个百姓未能受惠,也好像自己把他推入沟中一样。要普济万民,只有宰相能做到。现在签词说我当不了宰相,要实现利泽万民的心愿,莫过于当良医。如果真成为技艺高超的好医生,上可以疗君亲之疾,下可以救贫贱之厄,中能保身长全。身在民间而依旧能利泽苍生的,除了良医,再也没有别的了。"

Fan Zhongyan: Be a Loyal Minister or a Good Doctor

When Fan Zhongyan, a famous scholar in the Northern Song Dynasty, was still in obscurity and poverty, he once went to a temple to draw lots(bamboo slips used for divination), wishing to become the prime minister one day. But the slip words were negative. He drew again, praying that "If I can't be the prime minister, please let me be a good doctor." The slip was negative again. He then sighed and said, "The man who cannot benefit the people is not a real man."

One day somebody asked Fan, "It's reasonable for a man to have the aspiration to become a prime minister, but why are you praying to become a promising doctor. Isn't that inferior for you?"

Fan Zhongyan replied, "As a talented man, he should expect to help the rightful king to govern the country for the benefit of the people. He feels like being pushed into a pitch, if he can't benefit a single man. Only a prime minister can bestow benevolence to people all over the country. But if this position cannot be obtained, to become a doctor is the only way. A good doctor can treat the nobility and the common people. At least, he can keep fit for himself. No other occupation allows one to be so useful and noble."

钱乙自治

《宋史·方技》记载，北宋大医学家、"儿科之圣"钱乙，医术高超，但性情倔强。中年之后，他得了一种怪病，久治不愈，但还是坚持按自己的方式来治疗。后来病情加剧，他叹息着说："这种病就是'周痹啊，如果侵入内脏，就会死人的。我大概是要死了吧。"不久他又说："我可以把病转移到手脚上去。"于是自己制作药剂，日夜饮用。他的左手和左脚便突然间卷曲不能伸展了。他高兴地说："可以了！"

他的亲朋好友到东山采到了比斗还大的茯苓，他就按医方上的方法服用，直到把它吃完。这样他虽然半边手足偏废不能用，但髁骨节和健康人一样强壮。后来他以有病为理由，辞官回家，再也没有出过门。

钱乙处方用药时并不拘泥于某一师某一门。他什么书都读，对于古人的医疗方法也不拘泥、固执。他治病就像带兵打仗一样，经常安全地越过险要地带，故意暂时放纵敌人然后一举全歼，但结果又与医理吻合。他特别精通《本草》等书，分辨其中失误和遗缺的地方。有人找到奇怪罕见的药物，拿去问他，他总能说出该药的生长过程、形貌特点、名称和形状特征及与其他药的区别。把他说的拿回去与书对照，都能吻合。

晚年，他的瘫痪症状有所加剧，他知道自己治不好了，便把亲戚们找来告别，换好了衣服等待着死亡的来临，他就这样去世了，活到了82岁。

Qian Yi Healed Himself

According to the record in *Fang Ji of Song History*, Qian Yi（1032 –
1113）, the great medical scientist of the Northern Song Dynasty and the
Pioneer of Pediatic, had superb medical skills, but he was very stubborn. At
middle-age, he had a strange disease, which had been treated for a long time

but not healed yet. However, he insisted to treat it in his own ways. As the disease was aggravating, he sighed, "This disease is Zhou Bi. If it invaded into my viscera, I would be dead. I'm probably dying." Then he added : "I can move the disease to my hands and feet". So he made potions and drank them day and night. Suddenly, his left hand and left foot curled up and couldn't stretch. He said happily, "That's right!"

His relatives and friends went to Dong Mountain to pick up Fu Ling (tuckahoe), which was larger than a bucket, and he took it according to the doctor's guide until it was finished. In that way, although he couldn't use half of his hands and feet, his condyle was as strong as a healthy person's. Later, because of the disease, he resigned from office and never went outside.

When prescribing drugs, Qian Yi was not limited to a certain division. He read all books, and was unconstrained in using the medical methods of the ancients. In his treatment, like a general leading soldiers to war, he could cross the danger zone safely. He deliberately indulged the enemy temporarily, and then completely annihilated them, yet what he did conforms the medical theory. He was especially proficient in *Materia Medica*, and he could distinguish mistakes and missing parts. When people found some strange and rare herbs and went to him for answers. He could always tell their morphology, names and shapes, and the differences between this herb and others. What he said conforms to the medical classics.

In his later years, his symptoms of paralysis were aggravating and he knew that his days were numbered. So he said goodbye to his relatives, changed his clothes and waited for the death. He died at 82.

李时珍

　　李时珍是中国明代著名的医学家,他写了《本草纲目》一书。他所处的年代比牛顿要早一个多世纪。

　　当时有许多关于草药的书籍。但李时珍对这些书都不满意,因为书中有许多错误。有的草药定错了名,有的描述有错误,有的根本没有提到,所以他决定自己写一本书。

　　他坐下来写书之前,先四处采集草药,并对它们进行研究。他常常爬上高山,采集稀有的草药,就这样,他获得了一千多种草药的第一手资料,其中许多是前所未闻的。他还深入到劳动人民中间去,从他们那里学了许多东西。有一次,他看见有几个人正在熬煮粉红色的花。其中一个人对他说:"我们一年四季都在赶路,都有全身酸痛的病。我们熬煮的这种花叫作牵牛花,可以有效地止痛。"听到这么说,李时珍立刻记了下来。

　　一五七八年他最终完成了他的巨著。那时他已是六十岁的老人了。这本书他用了二十七年写成,是当时中国医学方面最好的一本书。

Li Shizhen

Li Shizhen(1518-1593)is a famous medical scientist of the Ming dynasty (1368-1644), who wrote *Compendium of Materia Medica*. The time he lived in was a century earlier than that of Newton.

At that time there were many books about herbs. But Li Shizhen was not satisfied with them, because there were too many mistakes. Some gave wrong names to the herbs, some gave the wrong descriptions, while others didn't give any description at all. So he decided to write a book himself.

Before he started writing, he went to many places to collect the herbs and made researches on them. He often climbed up to high mountains to collect rare herbs. In this way, he got the first-hand information about more than one thousand kinds of herbs, many of which haven't been heard of before. He also got close to farmers and learned many things from them. Once he saw several men boiling pink flowers. One of them told him, "You see, we are on the way all the year round, so we all have different sorts of aches in our body. The flower we are boiling is called morning glory and it's a perfect pain-killer." On hearing this, Li wrote down these words immediately.

Li finally finished his great work in 1578. By that time he was already in his sixties. It took him 27 years to write this book, which turned out to be the best book in medical science in China at that time.

喻嘉言救母子二人性命

　　说起古代的名医数不胜数,灿若星辰,他们有着高超的医术,往往能够救人于危难之际,成为老百姓的大救星。清代高士奇《牧斋遗事》记载了一个清初名医喻嘉言的故事。一天,他路过城北的一些破旧房子时,看到这里往往是居民临时停放棺材的地方。他突然看到一口好像是新停放的棺材底缝流出了鲜血。他急忙找到死者的丈夫,告诉他说:"你的妻子没有死。凡是人死了血色是黑暗的,活人的血色是鲜红的,我看见你妻子的棺材底流出的血是鲜红色的,快快开棺救治吧!"原来这位妇人因难产失血过多,昏迷后丈夫以为妻子死了,准备择期埋葬。喻嘉言诊妇人之脉,果然脉息未绝,于是就在她的心胸之间扎了一针,针还未拔出来,就听到呱呱的哭声。妇人分娩了,婴儿也得救了。她的丈夫背着复活的妻子,怀中抱着新生的婴儿,喜气洋洋地回家去了。

Yu Jiayan Saved Lives of the Mother and the Kid

There were countless celebrated doctors in ancient China who were as bright as the stars in the sky. They saved people's lives in time of difficulty and became known as the savior with their superb medical skills. The story of Yu Jiayan(1585-1670) , a famous doctor in the early Qing Dynasty, was recorded in *Mu Zhai Yi Shi* by Gao Shiqi(1645-1704) in the Qing Dynasty. One day, as he was passing through a district in the north of the city, he saw many coffins temporarily placed in the broken houses. He suddenly found blood dripping from the bottom of a new coffin. Yu told the dead woman's husband, "Your wife is still alive. The blood of the dead is dark while that of the living is bright red. I saw the blood from your wife's coffin is bright red! Open the coffin and let me save her!" It turned out that the woman had lost too much blood due to dystocia. Her husband thought his wife had passed away. Yu checked the woman's pulse and gave an acupuncture treatment for her. Before he pulled out the needle, he heard the crying from a newly-born baby. The woman gave birth to a baby and they were both saved. Her husband, carrying his resurrected wife and his son in his arms, went home joyfully.

叶天士治红眼病

清代名医叶天士治病颇有高招。一次,他遇上一位两眼通红的病人,病人眼眵堆满眼角,眼泪直往下淌,不断地用手去揩,露出十分忧虑的神情。叶天士见状,详细地询问病情,然后郑重地告诉病人说:"依我看,你的眼病并不要紧,只需吃上几帖药便会痊愈。严重的是你的两只脚底七天后会长出恶疮,那倒是一件麻烦事儿,弄不好有生命危险!"

病人一听,大惊失色,赶忙说:"好医生,既然红眼病无关紧要,我也没心思去治它了。请你快告诉我有什么办法渡过脚疮难关?"

叶天士思索良久,正色说道:"办法倒有一个,就怕你不能坚持。"病人拍着胸脯保证。于是叶天士向他介绍了一个奇特的治疗方案:每天用左手摸右脚底三百六十次,再用右手摸左脚底三百六十次,一次不能少,如此坚持方能渡过难关。

病人半信半疑,但想到这是名医的治法,便老老实实地照着做,七天后果然脚底没长出毒疮。更令他惊异的是:红眼病竟不知不觉地痊愈了。他高兴地向叶天士道谢,叶天士哈哈大笑,向他和盘托出,说道:"实话告诉你吧,脚底长毒疮是假的,我见你忧心忡忡,老是惦记着眼病,而你的眼疾恰恰与精神因素的关系很大,于是我想出这个办法,将你的注意力分散、转移到别处。除掉心病,眼疾便慢慢好了。"病人听完,惊奇不已,连声赞叹叶天士医术高明。

Ye Tianshi's Treatment for Pinkeyes

Ye Tianshi, a famous doctor of the Qing Dynasty, was very good at treating diseases. Once, he met a patient with pinkeyes which were full of discharge and tears running down his cheeks. Therefore, he wiped them with his hands all the time, showing an anxious look. Ye Tianshi observed the symptoms of the patient, and inquired about his illness in detail. Then he solemnly told the patient that his eye disease was not serious, and he required just taking some medicine for it. But the more serious problem was his feet that would threaten his life.

On hearing that, the patient was astonished and replied, "Since the pinkeye is not serious, I had no mind to treat it. Would you please tell me what to do with my feet?"

Ye Tianshi thought for a long time. Finally, he answered, "There is a way to treat your illness but I am afraid you can't persist". The patient patted his chest and made a promise. So Ye Tianshi introduced him to a special treatment: touching the bottom of the right foot 360 times with his left hand, and then touching the left foot 360 times with his right hand every day. As a result, he can pass through the difficulties.

Although the patient suspected, he did it as the doctor told him. Seven days later, the feet were safe. To his astonishment, the pinkeyes were imperceptibly healed. He expressed his gratitude to Ye Tianshi. But Ye Tianshi laughed and told him, "To tell you the truth, the poisoned sore was an excuse. I see you worried about your eye disease too much, which was greatly related to your mental factor. So I thought of this way to distract your attention. Then, the eye disease could be cured when you got rid of anxiety." The patient was surprised and praised repeatedly Ye Tianshi for his excellent medical skills.

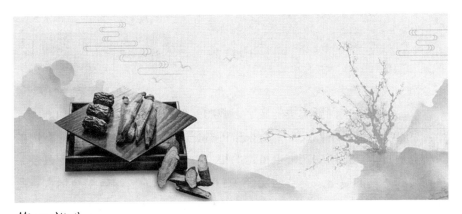

第二部分

Part Two

中草药的故事

Stories of Chinese Materia Medica

中草药

草药一直是中国药学史上文字记载的一部分,它的历史超过 4 000 年。相传,中国医药始于神农,一个传说中的神医。据说,他曾为了寻找有用的药材尝遍百草。中国中药采用植物的根、皮、花、种子、果实、叶、茎,以及来自动物和矿物的原料。当草药混合在一起时,它们的医疗效果会增大。此外,这些药物产生不良反应或副作用的风险较低。超过 3 000 种不同的草本植物被使用,但目前这些草药只有 300~500 种被普遍使用。

Chinese Herbal Medicine

Herbal medicine has been a part of the Chinese traditional medicine for over 4,000 years. According to legend, the Chinese herbal medicine was initiated by a legendary figure, Shennong. It is said that Shennong had tasted a hundred plants in a day in order to find useful medical herbs. Chinese herbal medicine employs roots, barks, flowers, seeds, fruits, leaves, and branches of the plant, as well as ingredients from animals and minerals. When herbs are mixed together, their medical effect increases. Moreover, the natural plants have a low risk of producing adverse reactions or side effects. Over 3,000 different herbs can be used, but only 300 to 500 of them are commonly used.

三七的故事

　　传说,有一次李时珍去南京参加药材展览会,在药王庙前的地摊上,看到一个云南药商摆着一种圆锥形褐黄色植物根,见过许多药材的李时珍也不认识这种药,便上前询问,药商说:"它叫三七,云南特产,可止血化瘀镇痛,是西南军队中治疗枪伤的重要药材。"李时珍取一细根头放入口中咀嚼,其味先苦后甜,凭借着往日的经验,觉得可带点回去一试,便问:"我买一两怎么样?"药商告诉他,这药的价格能和黄金相比,非常贵重,李时珍把钱袋里所有的钱拿出来都还不够,只得轻轻叹息一声,准备离开。

　　云南药商见他面善清瘦,身后跟着一个背着装有多种药材大包的青年,估计这是位对医药深有研究的人,便叫住他请教名字,李时珍说:"我叫李东璧。""啊,原来是蕲州李先生,久仰久仰! 今日有缘相见,荣幸荣幸! 我送你一两三七,愿你能为更多人治好病,也算是我的见面礼。"云南药商抓起几块三七递到李时珍手中。李时珍回去后取三七给好几个病人试用,效果非常好,他又从各个方面收集三七的治疗作用,将其载入《本草纲目》中。

The Story of Sanqi (Netoginseng Radix et Rhizoma)

As legend has it that Li Shizhen (1518 - 1593) once went to Nanjing to attend an exhibition of medicinal herbs. At a stall in front of the temple, he saw a druggist from Yunnan holding a cone-shaped brown-yellow plant root. Even Li Shizhen, who had seen many herbs, did not know about the drug. Then he asked the dealer. The dealer said, " It is called sanqi, a special product of Yunnan. It can stop blood stasis and relieve pain. It is an important herb for the southwest army to treat gunshot wounds. " Li Shizhen took a thin piece of the root and chewed it in his mouth. The taste was bitter first and sweet later. Thinking it might be worth a try, he asked, "What if I buy one *liang* (about 31. 25g) or two?" The druggist told him that the price of the medicine was as expensive as gold. Li Shizhen had not got enough money out of his purse, so he sighed softly and prepared to leave.

Seeing Li Shenzhen was a kind and thin young man with a large bag of various medicinal herbs on his back, the druggist thought that he might be a man who had an extensive knowledge of medicine. The druggist stopped him and asked for his name. Li Shizhen said, "My name is Li Dongbi." "Oh, are you Mr. Li from Qizhou? I've been looking forward to seeing you for a long time. It's my pleasure to meet you today. I'll give you one *liang* for free, and hope you can cure more people. It's also my gift to meet you." The Yunnan druggist picked up a few pieces of sanqi and handed them to Li Shizhen. Li went back to try sanqi on several patients and found that the effect was very good. He collected the therapeutic effect of this medicine from various aspects and put it into *the Compendium of Materia Medica*.

仙鹤草

古时有两个秀才进京赶考,途中路过一片沙滩地带。时值炎夏,烈日当空,晒得他们汗流浃背,又渴又累。这时,一个秀才流出鼻血,另一个慌了手脚,前不着村,后不着店,到哪里去寻药呢? 他们急中生智,用土块塞,用纸堵,但都无济于事,血又从鼻里流出来。

正在这时,忽然看见一只仙鹤嘴里衔着一根草,慢慢从头顶飞过来。他们想,如果我们也像仙鹤那样,长个翅膀,赶快飞走多好呀! 他俩用羡慕的口吻喊道:"仙鹤,仙鹤,慢慢飞呀,把你的翅膀借给我们用用,让我们赶快飞出这个鬼地方!"谁知仙鹤被他们这一叫,吓了一跳,把嘴一张,衔着的野草掉了下来。他们打趣地说:"翅膀借不下来,先拿野草润润嗓子吧。"流鼻血的秀才急忙把野草放在嘴里嚼了起来,有了水分的滋润,嗓子不干了,口也不渴了,过了一会儿,鼻血也不流了。他们高兴地急忙赶路。

后来,他们都中了进士,当了七品县官,就派人到山上找那种野草。经医生实践研究,证明这种野草确实有止血之效。为纪念送草的仙鹤,人们就把它取名叫"仙鹤草"。仙鹤草具有收敛止血、解毒疗疮、杀虫、涩汗、止咳、止血等功效,现代药理研究表明其具有抗肿瘤、抗炎、降血压等药理作用。

Crane Herb（Agrimoniae Herba）

In ancient times, two Xiucai(scholar who passed the imperial examination at the country level in the Ming and Qing Dynasties) went to the capital city to take the imperial examinations. When passing by a beach, they felt sweaty, thirsty and tired out in the sun. The worst of it, one of them got a nosebleed. The other was very flustered, "How can I find herbs in a desert land?" He just used paper or mud to plug the bloody nose. But it was useless to stop bleeding.

At this moment, a crane with a herb in its mouth flew overhead. They thought that if they were to have wings like cranes, they could fly away quickly. They said in an envious tone, "Crane, crane, fly slowly and give us your wings, so that we can get out of here very quickly." Unexpectedly, frightened by their sound, the crane opened its mouth and the herb was dropped to the ground. "Although we can't borrow the wings, we can use the herb to wet our thirsty throat," they said jokingly. The man with bleeding nose ate the herb quickly and his throat was no longer dry. After a while, nosebleeds were cured so they could continue their journey.

In the capital they were both successful in passing the exam and got some official positions. They asked some servants to go to the mountains to look for that kind of herb. Practical use shows that the herb has the function of stanching blood. Therefore, the herb is called "crane herb" to commemorate the crane's credit. Agrimony has the functions of astringent hemostasis, detoxification, killing pests, relieving sores, astringent sweat and cough, hemostasis and other effects. Modern pharmacological studies have shown that it has anti-tumor, anti-inflammatory and anti-hypertensive effects.

红景天

话说清代康熙年间,我国西部的巢望阿拉布坦发动叛乱,企图侵犯中原。为了平息叛乱,康熙御驾亲征。由于西部高原干旱,环境恶劣,加上官兵们长途跋涉,队伍劳顿,士气低落。在这样的情况下,部队战斗力大大减弱,屡屡战败。

在这关键时刻,幸好有一位老药农,将草药红景天给兵士们泡酒服用。结果大家体力恢复,士气大振,一鼓作气打败了叛军。于是,康熙给红景天取名"仙赐草",并把它钦定为御用贡品。从那时起,康熙打仗必带红景天。

Hong Jing Tian (Rhodiolae Crenulatae Radix et Rhizoma)

It is said that during the Kangxi period of the Qing Dynasty(1644−1911), a tribe named Tsewang Araptan in western China rebelled. They intended to invade the central plains. In order to suppress the rebellion, Emperor Kangxi led an army in person to fight the enemy. Due to the drought and bad environment of the western plateau, soldiers suffered a lot in the expedition. The morale of the army degenerated, and the fighting capacity was weakened, so they were defeated in battles. Luckily, a herb farmer gave a herb named Hong Jing Tian to the soldiers at this crucial moment. Soldiers soaked it in wine and drank it. Consequently, everybody was recovered and inspired. Finally they defeated the enemy and won the war. So, Kangxi named it "Magic Herb" and regarded it as a royal tribute. From then on, Kangxi took Hong Jing Tian with him whenever he went to war.

益母草

益母草可全草入药，有利尿消肿、收缩子宫的作用，是治疗妇科病的要药。关于益母草的来历，有一个小故事：

传说，程咬金的父亲因病早死，家里穷得叮当响。老母在生程咬金时，留下产后病。程咬金长大成人了，母亲的病还没有好，程咬金决心请郎中治好母亲的病。

为了给老母买药，程咬金一连几个晚上没睡觉工作，赚了一些钱到一个郎中的药铺，买了两剂中药。程母吃了草药，病情果然好转。程咬金高兴极了，又接连几个晚上没睡觉工作赚钱，去找那位郎中，可是，这位郎中说这次买的药得花更多钱。程咬金忽然灵机一动，就答应说："可以给你那么多钱，但要等我娘的病好了，再付你钱。"那位郎中同意了程咬金的要求。有一天，郎中到地里去采药，程咬金在后头跟着，偷看郎中采的是什么样的药，长在什么地方。后来，程咬金也到地里采郎中所采的那种药，煎汤给母亲治病，终于把母亲的病治好了。从此，程咬金就给这药草起了个名字，叫"益母草"。

Yi Mu Herb (Leonuri Herba)

Yi Mu Herb can be used in medicine and has a diuretic and uterotonic effect. It is an important Chinese medicine for the treatment of gynecological diseases. There goes a story about the origin of Lenourus.

It is said that General Cheng Yaojin's father died young due to an illness. The family was poor. His mother suffered from the postpartum disease after giving birth to Cheng Yaojin. When Cheng grew up, his mother was still sick. Cheng Yaojin decided to request a doctor to cure his mother's illness.

In order to buy medicine for his mother, Cheng worked several days and nights to earn money. He used the money to buy two doses of medicine from a drugstore. After taking the medicine, his mother got better. Cheng was so excited that he continued to work several days and nights for more money. He took the money to the doctor, only to be told that the medicine deserved more money. "Ok," he came up with an idea, "I'll give you the money when my mother fully recovers." The doctor agreed. One day, the doctor was gathering herbs in the fields, and Cheng followed him to see what kind of herb he picked up and where it grew. Later, Cheng went to the field to pick up the herb himself and boiled it for his mother. Finally, Cheng's mother got well. From then on, the medicine was designated by Cheng as Yi Mu Herb (meaning "good to the mother").

黄 连

从前,在土家族居住的黄水山上,有一位姓陶的名医。他家有个园子,专种药草,并用园中药草给人治病。由于医术高明,附近都有人来请他去治病。陶医生出门的时候多,就请了一个姓黄的帮工来管理园子。

陶医生的女儿叫妹娃,长得聪明、活泼,老两口视如掌上明珠。妹娃也喜欢栽花种药,每天早上起来,第一件事就是到园子里看花看药。

正月的一天早上,天气寒冷。妹娃沿着小路往山上走。忽然,她看到路边有一朵油绿色的小花开放了。妹娃越看越喜欢,就用手指把四周的泥土掏松,把它连根挖起,捧了回家,种在园子里。帮工看到这株在天寒地冻的正月也能开花的野花,也很喜欢,天天浇水,月月上肥。那草越长越茂盛,结了籽。帮工把这花的籽种在园子里,第二年,园里绿色的小花就开得更多了。

不料,妹娃得了一种怪病,浑身燥热,又吐又拉。只过了三天,她就瘦得只剩下皮包骨了。陶医生到外地给人治病尚未回来,妹娃的母亲只好请当地另一名医生前来给女儿治病。这是陶医生的朋友,诊治十分细心。可连服三剂药都未有好转,肚子越拉越厉害,还屙起血来。母亲整天守护在床前吃不下,睡不着,谈起女儿的病就掉泪。

帮工看在眼里,很焦急。忽然,他想起那绿色的小花,这种花草能不能做药呢?前个月自己喉咙痛,偶然摘下一片叶子,嚼了一下,虽然苦得要命,但过了一个时辰,喉咙痛居然减轻了。接着,他又嚼了两片叶子,当天就不痛了。妹娃这个病,不妨试一试呢?想到这里,他就连根带叶扯了一株起来,煎成一碗水,端给妹娃喝了。谁知早上喝的,下午病就好多了;再喝了两次,病居然全好了。这时,陶医生回来了,一问经过,感动得握着帮工的手,连声感谢,说:"妹娃害的是肠胃热病,一定要清热解毒的药才医得好。这开绿花的小草,看来对清热解毒有特效呀!"

这位帮工姓黄名连,为了感谢他,这药材也就定名为"黄连"了。

Huang Lian (Coptidis Rhizoma)

Once upon a time, on Mount Huangshui where the ethnic Tujia people lived, there was a famous doctor surnamed Tao. He was specialized in treating people with herbs planted in his garden. Because of his excellent medical skills, he was invited to see patients nearby. When Dr. Tao went out, Huang, a housework helper was hired to run his garden.

Meiwa, Dr. Tao's daughter, was clever and lively. The old couple regarded her as the apple of the eye. Meiwa liked to plant flowers and herbs, too. Every morning when she got up, the first thing she did was to go to the garden to look at the flowers and herbs.

On one cold morning in January of lunar calendar, the little girl walked up the hill along the path. Suddenly, she saw a little green flower blossoming by the roadside. The more she looked at it, the more she liked it. She dug up the soil around and picked it up with her fingers. She took it home and planted it in the garden. Since it was blossoming in the frozen and cold January, their housework helper Huang also liked it very much. He watered and fertilized it. The flower grew more and more luxuriant and became seeded. Huang planted the seed of the flower in the garden, and the next year the little green flower in the garden bloomed even more.

Unexpectedly, Meiwa got a strange disease. Feeling hot and dry, she had vomiting and diarrhea. Only after three days, she was nothing but skin and bones. Dr. Tao was on his business and had not come back yet. Her mother had to ask another doctor to treat her daughter. This doctor, Tao's friend, was very careful but no effect was seen after three doses of medicine. The diarrhea became even more severe, having blood in one's stool. The mother took care of her all day without eating or sleeping. She couldn't help crying when talking about her daughter's illness.

Huang was anxious to see what had happened. Suddenly he remembered the little green flower. Could this flower be used as medicine? When he had a sore throat last month, he picked up a leaf by chance and chewed it. It was very bitter, but after an hour, the sore throat was relieved. Then he chewed two more leaves and the pain subsided on that day. Could Meiwa have a try as well? Thinking of it, he took it up with roots and leaves, boiled it into a bowl of water and served Meiwa. Unexpectedly, she was much better in the afternoon. After drinking twice, she was all right. At this time, Dr. Tao came back. When he knew that, he was so moved that he held his helper's hand and thanked him repeatedly, "Meiwa got intestinal and stomach fever and the medicine must be used to clear away heat and toxic substances. This little green flower seems to have special effects on clearing away heat and toxic substances."

In order to thank him, the medicinal herb was named Huanglian, Huang's full name.

断肠草(钩吻)

相传神农经常帮助周围的人解决一些难题。为了寻找能缓解人们疾病苦痛的药材,他常年到深山老林中遍尝百草,哪怕中毒也在所不惜。

有一天神农看到一些翠绿的叶子而且有淡淡的香味,于是摘下一片服下。可是意想不到的是,当食用了这片叶子后,他感觉胃肠变得特别清爽。于是神农就将这种叶子常常带在身边以便解毒之用。

自那以后当尝试毒草后感觉不舒服,神农就立即吞这种叶子,神农尝试了很多有毒的植物,都能化险为夷。直到有一次,神农在一个向阳的地方发现了一种叶片相对而生的藤,这种藤上开着淡黄色的小花,于是神农就摘了片叶子放进嘴里咽下。可是令他意想不到的是毒性很快发作,出现了一些不适之感。神农马上吞下那种解毒的叶子,却感觉自己的肠子已经断成一截一截的了,不多久,这位尝近无数草药的神农,就这样断送了自己的性命,因此这种植物也被人们称为断肠草。

"断肠草"又称为"钩吻"。钩吻有显著的镇痛作用和催眠的作用。目前,"钩吻"的药用价值已在我国许多领域广泛应用。

Intestines-broken Herb (Geldrmium Elegans)

According to the legend, Shennong often helped people to solve their problems. In search of the medicinal herbs to relieve the pain of the people, he went into the mountains and forests year after year to taste medicinal herbs even if they were poisonous.

One day, Shennong saw a few green leaves with faint fragrance and picked up a piece of it to have a taste. He was surprised to find that his stomach and intestines were especially refreshing. Therefore, Shennong often carried the leaves with him for detoxification.

Since then, every time he felt uncomfortable after eating a poisonous plant, he chewed and swallowed up the leaves immediately. He tried many poisonous plants, but fortunately, he was always able to get himself out of danger by chewing these leaves. One day, in a sunny area, Shennong found a kind of rattan yellow symmetric flowers. He took off a piece of the leaves and swallowed it up. But to his unexpectation, his organism was quickly attacked by the toxicity of the leaf and he felt uncomfortable soon. Shennong immediately swallowed the detoxified leaf, but it was too late, his intestines had been broken into pieces. What a regret! Shennong, who had tasted hundreds of herbs, died in this way. Later people named the plant as intestines-broken herb.

Intestines-broken herb is also called Gou Wen. Its functions include remarkable analgesic and hypnotic effect. At present, the medicinal value of gelsemium elegans has been widely used in many fields in our country.

夏枯草

从前有位书生叫茂松，为人厚道，自幼攻读四书五经，然而却屡试不第。茂松因此终日郁闷，天长日久，积郁成疾，颈部长出许多瘰疬（即淋巴结核），如蚕豆般大小，形似链珠，有的溃破流脓。久医无效，病情越来越重。

这年夏天，茂松爹不远千里寻神农。一日，他来到一座山下，只见遍地绿草茵茵，似入仙境。他刚想歇息，不料昏倒在地。

茂松爹怎么也没有料到，这百草如茵的仙境，竟是神农的药圃。此时，神农正在给药草浇水施肥，见有人晕倒急忙赶来救治。茂松爹醒来，谢恩并诉说了自己的苦衷。神农听罢，从草苑摘来药草，说："用此草上端球状部分，煎汤服用。"又说："此草名'夏枯草'，夏天枯黄时采集入药，有清热散结之功效。"茂松按方服之，不久病愈。后来，父子二人广种夏枯草，为民治病，深得人心。

The Story of Xiaku Grass (Prunellae Spica)

Once upon a time, there was a scholar named Mao Song, who was kind to everyone. He studied *The Four Books* and *The Five Classics* since young but failed several times in the imperial examinations. Therefore, Mao Song was depressed all day. As time went by, he got an illness that he had a lot of lymph nodes in the neck, which were about the size of the horsebeans and shaped like a chain of beads. Some of them were broken, letting out of pus. Long-term treatment had no effect and his condition was from bad to worse.

In that summer, in order to cure his son's disease, Mao Song's father traveled thousands of miles in an effort to find Shennong. One day, he came to the foot of a mountain where green grasses grew everywhere, and the scene looked like a fairyland. He was about to take a break but fainted to the ground unconsciously.

By chance, the grassy fairyland was actually the medicinal garden of Shennong. At that moment, Shennong found Mao Song's father collapsed on the ground while he was watering and fertilizing the herbs. So he rushed over to give him a treatment. Mao Song's father woke, thanked Shennong and told him why he came here. After listening to the father's words, Shennong picked some herb from his medicinal garden and said, "You use the ball-shaped part of the grass to boil water for your son." Shennong added, "This grass is called Xiaku Grass, collected in summer when the leaves turn yellowish. It has the effect of clearing away heat and reducing swelling. Taking the medicine back, Mao Song's father did as Shen Nong told him. Mao Song got healthy soon. Afterwards, Mao Song and his father planted Xiaku Grass (selfheal) on a large scale and used it to treat people who had the same disease. People were all grateful to them and Shennong.

鱼腥草

　　当年,越王勾践做了吴王夫差的俘虏,勾践忍辱负重假意百般讨好夫差,方被放回越国(今绍兴)。传说勾践回国的第一年,越国碰上了罕见的荒年,百姓无粮可吃。为了和百姓共渡难关,勾践翻山越岭终于寻找到一种可以食用的野菜,而且生长能力特别强,总是割了又长,生生不息。于是,越国上下竟然靠着这小小的野菜渡过了难关。这种野菜有鱼腥味,被勾践命名为"鱼腥草"。

　　现代药理实验表明,鱼腥草具有抗菌、抗病毒、提高机体免疫力、利尿等作用。

Yu Xing Cao (Houttuyniae Herba)

In the Spring and Autumn Period (770 B.C. – 476 B.C.), Gou Jian, the King of Yue, was captured by Wu. He pretended to please the king of Wu, Fu Chai. Finally, he was released to Yue (now Shaoxing). Unfortunately, famine broke out in the first year he returned. To tide over the disaster, Gou Jian found an edible wild herb in the mountains after innumerable trials and hardships. The wild herb grew rapidly and helped the local people get through the difficulty. The wild herb smelled and tasted like raw fish (pinyin: Yu). Therefore, Gou named it "Yu Xing Cao".

According to modern pharmacological experiments, houttuynia cordata has the effects of resisting bacteria and virus, improving immunization and promoting diuresis.

金银花

相传很久以前,在江南某山区,住着一对老夫妻,靠开药店为生,膝下有一女,长得如花似玉,人们叫她金银花。

金银花从小跟随父母配药方,懂得许多药理知识。有一年,村里闹瘟疫,不少人被病魔夺去了生命。金银花见乡亲们遭此磨难,决心寻找灭瘟方,几番试验,终于配成一种"避瘟汤"。

这时有户权贵人家看中金银花,要给傻儿子说亲,并扬言:"如若不允,休想开药店!"金银花秉性刚烈,以死相抗。乡亲们感谢金银花的恩德,把她葬在风景秀丽的山冈上。次年,坟上长出一簇簇金黄、银白相间的鲜花,分外妖娆,人们叫它金银花。

金银花清热解毒,疏散风热。

现代治疗中常用于风热感冒,温病发热。

Jin Yin Flower (Lonicerae Japonicae Flos)

Long long ago, there was an old couple, who ran a drugstore for a living in a mountainous region in the south of the Yangtze River. Their only daughter was as pretty as the Jin Yin Flower(meaning "gold and silver flower"), so she was called Jinyinhua.

When she was a little girl, the girl learned to make prescriptions from her parents and knew many pharmacological knowledge. One year, a serious plague outbroke and many people were killed by the disease. The girl saw the local folks' suffering, determined to find out a medicine that could cure the disease. After repeated tests, she invented the "Bi Wen Decoction"(meaning "soup to evade the plague").

Meanwhile, a rich household wanted her to marry their silly son and threatened that, "The drugstore must be closed if she refused!" Jinyinhua was unyielding and resisted with her life. The villagers thanked her and buried her in a beautiful hillside. The following year, clusters of gold and silver flowers grew around her grave, which were more enchanting and blooming. So, people called it "Jin Yin Flower".

Jin Yin Flower (Honeysuckle) can clear away heat and toxic substances, and disperse wind heat. It is usually used to cure wind heat and cold and febrile disease in modern clinic.

茵　陈

相传,有一个黄痨病人(黄疸),面色姜黄,眼睛凹陷,极度消瘦,找到华佗:"先生,请你给我治治病吧。"华佗皱着眉摇了摇头说:"眼下医生们还没有找到治疗黄痨病的办法,我也是无能为力呀!"

半年后,华佗又碰见那个病人,发现他变得非常健康,身体强壮,满面红润。华佗大吃一惊,急忙问道:"你这病是哪位医生治好的?"

那人回答道:"我没请医生看,病是自己好的。"

华佗不信:"哪有这种事!你准是吃了什么药吧?"

"药倒没有吃过,不过因为春荒没粮,我吃过些野草。"

"这就对了!草就是药,你吃了多少天?"

"一个多月。"

"吃的什么草啊?"

他们走到山坡上,那人指着一片绿茵茵的野草说:"就是这个。"

华佗一看是青蒿,便采了一些,给其他黄痨病人试服,但试了几次,均无效果。华佗又问那人,吃的几月的蒿,病人说是三月的。华佗醒悟到,春三月百草发芽,也许三月蒿子有药力。

第二年春天,华佗又采了许多三月的青蒿,给黄痨病人服用,果然吃一个好一个。为摸清青蒿的药性,第三年,华佗把根、茎、叶分类试验,发现只有幼嫩的茎叶可以入药治病,并取名"茵陈"。

Yin Chen (Artemisiae Scopariae Herba)

A man, who suffered from jaundice, had a ginger face, hollow eyes and a skinny body, said to Hua Tuo, " Doctor Hua, please help me." Hua Tuo frowned his brows and shook his head, "There is no treatment for such a disease.

I can do nothing for it."

Half a year later, Hua Tuo met the man again. Surprisingly, the man became very healthy with a strong body and a ruddy face. Then, Hua Tuo asked him in eager, "Could you tell me who cured your disease?"

"Nobody. It was self-healing."

"That's impossible. You must have taken some medicine." Hua Tuo said.

"I never took any medicine, but I ate some herbs in the spring famine."

"That's it. The herbs are equal to medicine. How long have you had those herbs?"

"More than one month."

"What kind of herb did you eat?"

They walked to the hillside, and then the man pointed to a green grass weeds and said, "That's it."

Hua Tuo picked up some of this herb and tried to cure other patients who suffered from jaundice. But it turned out to be ineffective. Then Hua Tuo asked the man again, "When did you eat the herds?"

"In March."

Hua Tuo realized that the plant sprouted in March every year. Maybe only the sweet wormwood in March had the effect.

Hua Tuo picked up sweet wormwood next spring, gave those patients to eat, and then all the patients were cured.

In the third year, Hua Tuo picked up more sweet wormwood and dried it for use. Experiments showed that only the young stems and leaves of the sweet wormwood had the efficacy. He named it as "Yin Chen".

吴茱萸

据说,"吴茱萸"在春秋时候原名"吴萸"。它产在吴国,是一味止痛良药。

当时,吴国和邻近的楚国相比,还算小国,小国就得向大国进贡。

这一年,吴国的贡品之中就有吴萸。谁想楚王一见,竟大发雷霆:"小小的吴国,胆敢把以国命名的东西当贡品,这不是看不起堂堂的楚国吗?拿回去,不收!"吴国的使者愣住了。

这时,有位姓朱的楚国大夫,急忙对楚王说:"吴萸能治胃寒腹疼,还能止吐止泄。吴王听说大王有腹痛的老病,才选来进贡的。如果拒绝接受,那不就伤了两国的和气吗?""胡说,"楚王喝道,"我用不着什么'吴萸'!我们的国家也不需要!"吴国的使臣又羞又气,退出王宫。朱大夫追出来说:"请你不要生气。就把吴萸留给我吧。楚王早晚会用上它的。"吴使就把吴萸给了朱大夫。朱大夫拿到家中,栽在院内,还命人精心护理。吴使回国后,吴王一听楚王这么无礼,就同楚国断了交。

几年过后,吴萸在朱大夫家中长得枝繁叶茂,已经有一大片了。朱大夫知道,这种草的果实需在未成熟的时候入药;所以,他命人及时采摘,晾干收藏,保存了许多。有一天,楚王忽然旧病复发,肚子痛得直冒虚汗。朝中的大夫都急坏了,可是谁也没有办法治。朱大夫急忙用吴萸煎汤,献给楚王。楚王连吃了几剂,肚子不痛了;再吃几剂,病全好了。楚王就问朱大夫:"你给我送来的是什么药啊?"朱大夫说:"这就是那个吴国进贡的吴萸。"这时,楚王才后悔不该那样对待吴国。他一面派人与吴国和好,一面命人大种吴萸。

有一年秋天,楚国流行起瘟病来了。许多百姓上吐下泻,有的甚至活活病死了。楚王急忙传旨,命令朱大夫配药救民。朱大夫以吴萸为主制药,救活了许多快死的病人。楚王为让人们记住朱大夫的功劳,就传旨把"吴萸"更名为"吴朱萸"。

后来,人们为了标明这是一种草,又把"吴朱萸"的"朱"字,加了草头,写成了"吴茱萸"。

Wu Zhu Yu (Euodiae Fructus)

It is said that Wu Zhu Yu (Evodia) was originally called Wu Yu in the Spring and Autumn Period(770 B.C.–476 B.C.). Produced in Wu State, it was a medicine for pain-relieving.

At that time, compared to the neighboring Chu State, Wu was still a small country. Small countries had to pay tribute to superpower countries.

One year, Wu Yu, as the tribute of Wu, was sent to Chu. Surprisingly, the King of Chu was more than furious at the tribute. "How dare Wu take the thing named after the state as a tribute! Is it a disdain to our dignified Chu? Take it back! I do not accept it!" The emissary of Wu was stunned.

At this moment, Doctor Zhu of Chu hurried to explain to the king, "Wu Yu can not only cure stomach cold and abdomen pain, but also stop vomiting and diarrhea. The king of Wu heard that Your Majesty had problems of diarrhea, so they chose it as a tribute. If you refuse to accept it, I am afraid this will harm the relationship of our two countries." "Nonsense!" The king of Chu said, "I don't need Wu Yu and our country doesn't need it either!" Then the emissary of Wu felt a shamed and had to leave. At this moment, Doctor Zhu chased out and talked to the emissary, "please don't be furious. Just leave Wu Yu to me. The king of Chu will understand your sincerity one day." So the emissary of Wu gave Wu Yu to Doctor Zhu. Doctor Zhu took it home, planted it in the courtyard, and ordered his servants to look after it carefully. The emissary returned to his homeland and told the king what had happened in Chu. The king of Wu decided to break off diplomatic relations with Chu after listening to his description.

A few years later, Wu Yu grew luxuriantly in Doctor Zhu's backyard. Doctor Zhu knew that the fruit of this kind needed to be put into medicine when immature, so he ordered his servants to pick and dry the collection in time and store a lot.

One day, the king of Chu got sick again, and he had severe stomach pain and abnormal sweating.

All doctors were anxious, but no one could cure it. Doctor Zhu sent Wu Yu to the king. After a few doses, the pain stopped. And a few doses more, he was fine. The king asked Doctor Zhu, "What medicine did you send to me?" Zhu said, "This is Wu Yu presented by Wu." At this time, the king regretted that Wu should not be treated like that. He sent people to restore the relationship with Wu, and ordered servants to plant Wu Yu on a large scale.

In the autumn of a year, a seasonal febrile disease began to spread in Chu. Many people got vomit and diarrhea, and some even died. The king of Chu gave order to Doctor Zhu to save people's life. Doctor Zhu used Wu Yu as the main medicine and saved quite a lot dying patients. The king of Chu hoped that people could remember Doctor Zhu's credit, so he ordered that "Wu Yu" was renamed "Wu Zhu Yu".

Afterwards, people marked it as a kind of herb and added the component "Zhu" between "Wu" and "Yu". It was written as "Wu Zhu Yu".

辛　夷

秦举人得了一种怪病,鼻孔流脓流涕,腥臭难闻。这种病很讨人嫌,连他的妻子儿女也躲得远远的。秦举人请过许多医生,但吃什么药都没用。他想:这么活着招人嫌恶还不如死了好,就打算寻死。有个朋友知道后劝道:"天下这么大,本地医生治不好,何不到外边求医去? 还能顺便逛逛名山大川,散散心。"

秦举人一听有理,反正待在家里也尽跟老婆孩子呕气,于是带了个家人,骑着马出门了。

秦举人走了很多地方,他走到南方的一个夷族人居住的地区,有个夷家医生说:"这病好治。"

秦举人喜出望外,急忙请他医治。

医生到山上采了一种花苞回来,让秦举人服用,秦举人吃了半个月,鼻子真的不流脓了。他十分高兴,对医生说:"这种药真灵,你能不能让我带一些回去,万一再犯病时就不用跑这么远求医了。"

医生想了想说:"不如给你带些种子回去栽种。"

秦举人更加高兴,他重重酬谢了医生,带着种子回家了。到家后,他就种植这种草药。几年过后,院子里长了一大片。凡有人得了鼻病,他就用这种草药给人医治。

人们问:"这药草叫什么名字?"

秦举人一想,忘了问夷家医生了。又一想,这是在辛亥年间从夷人那里引来的,就说:"这叫'辛夷吧!"

辛夷的功效是发散风寒通鼻窍,临床多用于风寒感冒,是治鼻渊、鼻塞流涕的要药。

Xin Yi (Magnoliae Flos)

Qin, a Juren (scholar who had passed the imperial exam at provincial level), had a strange disease. His nose was mattery and smelt bad. This kind of illness made him disgusted by his neighbors, and even his wife and daughter fought shy of him. Mr. Qin went to see many doctors, but no one could cure it. For these reasons, he felt so upset that he decided to commit suicide. Mr. Qin's friend learned that and said, "The world is very wide. since local doctors can't cure you, why not go out to see a doctor? At the same time, you can also go travelling and relaxing."

Qin agreed, rode on a horse and went out with a servant.

Several days later, he came to an area in the south inhabited by Yi nationality. A Yi doctor said, "Don't worry, this is a small case."

Mr. Qin was very happy and asked the doctor to treat him at once.

The doctor went to the hills and gathered a kind of buds to treat Qin's disease. Half a month later, his nose got well. He was so happy that he asked the doctor if he could bring some medicine back so that he could cured himself without going so far.

The doctor thought for a while and said, "Why don't you bring some seeds back to plant?"

Mr. Qin was more pleased, so he rewarded the doctor and went home with the seeds. He planted this herb as soon as he got home. A few years later, a large piece of this herb had been grown up in the yard. So long as anyone had nasal disease, he gave this herb to him.

Someone asked, "What's the name of this herb?"

Mr. Qin forgot to ask the Yi doctor about the name of this herb. But, this herb was from the Yi doctor at Xin Hai year, so he said, "This herb is called Xin Yi."

The effect of Xin Yi is diverging cold and relieving nose. It is used for the treatment of cold in clinic. And it is an important medicine that treats cold, nasal obstruction and running nose.

鹅不食草

鹅不食草味辛性温,归肺经,具有发散风寒,通鼻窍,止咳,解毒,止痒等功效。下面是关于它的来历的故事。

从前,有一个农家的孩子,自幼患鼻炎,长年鼻塞流黄脓鼻涕,臭烘烘的。孩子家里养有一群鹅,一天,他赶着鹅群到一个山边的地方吃草。饿坏了的鹅群见草就吃,唯独有一种又鲜又嫩的青草,鹅群却一口都不吃。小孩用竹竿把鹅群赶到草旁,鹅群只低头闻闻,又跑开了。小孩心里好奇,拔一株草用鼻子闻了一会儿,忽然打了几个喷嚏,鼻子顿时通畅了。于是,小孩天天赶鹅群来这里放养,同时天天嗅闻这种青草,后来,小孩再也不流浓鼻涕了。同村还有几个患鼻炎的孩子,也用这种青草治鼻塞,都很快治愈了。从此,这种草的药用功效逐渐流传开。因为鹅不肯吃这种草,因此人们就给它取名为"鹅不食草"。

Goose-Not-Eat Grass (Centipedae Herba)

According to Chinese medicine, Goose-Not-Eat Grass (Centipeda minima) tastes warm and spicy, belonging to the lung channel. It can dissipate wind-cold, free nasal orifices, and relieve coughing, detoxification and itching. Here goes a story about its origin.

Once upon a time, there was a kid who had rhinitis since childhood. He had a stuffed nose and the yellow snivel ran down his nose with foul smell. The child's family raised a flock of geese. One day, he was tending the goose on a hillside. The hungry geese ate the tender grass whenever they saw, but they fought shy of a kind of grass which was fresh and tender. The kid drove the geese to the grass again by a bamboo stick, but the geese just smelt it and ran away. The kid was inquisitive, so he smelt the grass. Suddenly he sneezed, and his nose was no longer obstructed. From then on, the kid drove the geese here every day and sniffed this kind of grass at the same time. Before long, the kid got rid of the thick mucus. Other children who suffered from rhinitis in the village were also treated with this kind of grass. Since then, the medicinal efficacy of this grass was gradually known to people. Because the goose doesn't eat this grass, people named it Goose-Not-Eat Grass.

薏苡明珠

马援奉令去南疆（今广东、广西等地）平定叛乱。马援在交州时就常食用薏苡的种仁——薏米，认为它能"轻身省欲，以胜瘴气"。薏苡是一味中药，也可食用，具有健脾、补肺、清热、利湿之功。南方的薏苡仁大而优，马援在班师回朝时，就特意带回了一车薏苡籽，准备用作种子来种植。由于薏苡籽实呈球形，外包有似珐琅质的硬壳，看上去确实有点像珍珠。朝中的一些权贵就认为马援车中装的是私掠的明珠等珍宝。由于马援当时很受光武帝的重用，这般权贵们不敢有所动作。等到马援死后，监军梁松嫉贤妒能，就上书诬告马援搜刮了大量的明珠宝物，归为己有。汉光武帝竟然相信了这些不实之辞，龙颜大怒，传旨追回马援的"新息侯印"，使马援的妻子马夫人不敢报丧，偷偷的把马援的棺材埋在城外，连以前宾客故人也不敢上马家吊丧。后世以"薏苡明珠""薏苡之谤"比喻忠良蒙冤被谤。

Yiyi（Coicis Semen）

Ma Yuan was ordered to go to the south（now Guangdong, Guangxi, etc.）to suppress a rebel. He used to eat Job's Tear（coix seed）when he stationed in Jiaozhou. The seed has the effect of lossing weight and suppressing miasma. Coix is both a Chinese medicine and an edible food. It can strengthen spleens, tonify lungs, and clear away heat and dampness. Coix seeds in the south are especially fine. When Ma won the war and went back to the capital, he deliberately brought back a car of coix seeds. The seed looked like pearls, round with an enamel-like hard shell. Some people in the court thought that they were pearls and jewels grabbed by Ma in the south. At that time, since the king Guangwu thought highly of Ma, those influential officials dare not say anything bad about

Ma. When Ma died, Liang Song, a military inspector, was jealous of Ma's virtue and wrote a report to the emperor, saying that Ma had grabbed a lot of pearls and jewelry from the poor and had not handed in to the court. The king was so furious that he with drawed Ma's official title "Xinxi Hou". Ma's wife did not report the news of his funeral and buried him outside the city secretly. All Ma's friends did not go to Ma's house to express their condolences. After that, "coix pearl" and "coix slander" slander are used as a metaphor for people who are defamed by false charges.

石菖蒲

相传,在公元 1144 年,20 岁的南宋大诗人陆游与舅舅的女儿唐琬结婚。婚后夫妻感情甚佳。没想几个月后,唐琬却患了尿频症,一昼夜排尿20 多次,整个人被折磨得形销神脱,痛苦异常。陆游十分着急,遍寻医生诊治,却总不见效。一天,已成名医的好友郑樵来访,诊察病情后,开了张处方,将石菖蒲、黄连各等份,研为细末,每天早晚各以黄酒冲服 6 克。唐琬服了没几天,病竟豁然痊愈。陆游十分感谢郑樵,也对石菖蒲赞誉有加,挥毫写下脍炙人口的《菖蒲》诗。

石菖蒲性味辛温,归心、胃经,具有醒神益智和化湿开胃的功效。

Shi Chang Pu (Acori Tatarinowii Rhizoma)

According to legend, Lu You, a famous poet in the Southern Song Dynasty (1127 – 1279) , married his uncle's daughter, Tang Wan, when he was 20 years old in 1144. After the marriage, the young couple lived happily. However, a few months later, Tang Wan suffered from a disease—frequent urination, which tortured her so much that she became weak and pained. Lu You was so worried that all the doctors could do nothing for her. One day, Zheng Qiao, a friend of Lu You, who was also a famous doctor, dropped in and wrote him a prescription including calamus, coptis chinensis and yellow wine. Tang's illness gradually recovered a few days later after taking Zheng's medicine. Lu was more than grateful to Zheng Qiao, so he wrote the famous poem *Calamus*.

Calamus is a warm-natured herb and works for heart and stomach meridian. It has the function of awakening mind, resolving dampness and stimulating appetite.

豆蔻年华

　　豆蔻,多年生常绿草本植物,产于岭南。高丈许,外形像芭蕉,叶大,披针形,淡黄色,秋季结实,果实扁球形,种子像石榴子,可入药,有香味。可用于化湿消痞,行气温中,开胃消食。用于湿浊中阻,不思饮食,湿温初起,胸闷不饥,寒湿呕逆,胸腹胀痛,食积不消。

　　杜牧的赠别诗中的句子"娉娉袅袅十三余,豆蔻梢头二月初。春风十里扬州路,卷上珠帘总不如。"杜牧用含苞待放的一朵豆蔻花来形容女子十三岁的年纪,比喻贴切而形象,迅速被世人传颂,以至于生活中人们常说的豆蔻的本意已基本消失,现在豆蔻一般指十三四岁的女子,代指少女的青春年华。

Budding Beauty (Amomi Fructus Rotundus)

Cardamom, a kind of perennial evergreen herb, grows in the southern area of China. The plant looks like banana, several meters tall with big yellow leaves. It usually bears fruits in the fall. Its flat globose fruit looks like pomegranate with fragrance which can be used as medicine to resolve dampness, eliminate pathogens, activate *qi*, warm the middle-*jiao* (portion of the body housing the stomach and spleen) and stimulate the appetite. It can be used to treat damp-caused middle impedance, loss of appetite, the beginning of the damp-warm, chest distress, cold-dampness-caused emesia, chest and belly swelling pain and indigestion. There is a poem by Du Mu, a great poet in the Tang Dynasty, comparing a 13-year-old girl to a budding cardamom flower:

She is slender and graceful and not yet fourteen,

Like a cardamom at the tip of a new spray.

The vernal wind uprolls the pearly window-screen,

Her face outshines those on the splendid three-mile way.

(Tr. X.Y. Z)

This metaphor was soon spreading far and near for its aptness and vividness. Nowadays the cardamom is usually used to describe girls between 13 and 14 years old while the original meaning of cardamom is basically missing.

徐长卿

　　话说赵匡胤大权在握，终日饮酒作乐，以致酒色伤身。经不少御医诊治，总是难以治愈。一日，徐长卿看见宋太祖脸色异常，手顶胃区，甚感痛苦，忙前去探问。一问才知道皇上酗酒伤胃，老胃病又复发了。徐长卿从小学过医道，略懂一些中医药知识。于是，去野外采集一味草药，煎水给赵匡胤服用。谁知，这味药还真管用，很快皇上的顽疾竟神奇地解除了。

　　皇上很惊奇地说："御医都无奈，你怎有如此医技，此药叫什么名字？"徐长卿答道："皇上，臣有无礼之罪，此药还没有名字呢。"赵匡胤闻言道："爱卿，你叫徐长卿，这药就以你的名字命名吧！"从此，这种中草药有了一个叫徐长卿的药名了。

　　现代药理研究表明：徐长卿主含丹皮酚、黄酮甙和少量生物碱，具有镇痛、镇静、抗菌、降压、降血脂等作用。对骨伤科的跌打损伤、腰椎痛、胃炎、胃痛、胃溃疡等引起的胃脘胀痛均有十分显著的止痛效果。难怪宋太祖的老胃病被治愈。徐长卿这味中药现今被列为祛风湿药，也是民族医药十分钟爱的止痛祛风除湿和解蛇毒之药，一直被广泛使用。

Xu Changqing（Cynanchi Paniculati Radix et Rhizoma）

　　Zhao Kuangyin, Emperor of the Song Dynasty(927-976), was addicted to drinking and sex day and night, resulting in damages to his health. Though treated by quite a few imperial doctors, his sickness couldn't be cured. One day, Xu Changqing, a doctor of traditional Chinese medicine, saw that the emperor seemed to have an abnormal face and pain in the stomach area. Xu Changqing hurried to inquire him. Through the conversation, Xu knew that the Emperor was having abdominal pain due to excessive drinking, his gastric disease relapsed again. Having learned traditional Chinese medicine since childhood, Xu knew some Chinese herbs. Therefore, he collected a handful of a herb in the field and boiled it for the Emperor. Unexpectedly, the herb worked and eliminated the disease of the emperor quickly.

The emperor said surprisingly, "The imperial doctors were helpless at my gastric disease, how did you succeed in treating it? What's the name of the herb?" Xu replied, "The herb has no name yet, Your Majesty." Zhao said, "Your name is Xu Changqing, and I will make the herb be named after you!" Since then, this kind of Chinese medical herb has its name as Xu Changqing.

It's shown by modern pharmacological research that Xu Changqing mainly contains paeonol, flavonoid glycoside and a small amount of alkaloids which has many functions such as analgesia, sedation, antimicrobial, antihypertensive and antilipidemic effect. It has significant painrelief effects on the traumatic injury of bone, the lumbar pain and gastric abscess caused by gastritis, stomach ache and gastric ulcer. No wonder the emperor's old stomach trouble was cured. Xu Changqing is now listed as an antirheumatic Chinese herb. It has been widely used to relieve pain, dispel wind and eliminate dampness and can also be used to cure snakebites in the folk medicine.

人　参

从前,在东北山村,有一对兄弟,于冬天带上弓箭、皮衣和干粮上山去打猎。上山的第二天,狂风大作、雪花纷飞,大雪下了三天三夜,山路全被大雪覆盖,迷了路的兄弟俩无法出山。他们找了棵空心大树藏身,为了节约粮食,又挖些草根充饥。偶然发现有一种大拇指粗的草根,形状像人的胳膊和腿,放到嘴里一尝,甜津津的,吃了这东西,他们感到浑身更有劲了,有时吃多了还会流鼻血。因此,他们每天就只吃一点儿。

直到第二年开春,兄弟俩才满载着猎物下山回家。村里的人以为他俩早死了,见他们又白又胖地回来,都奇怪地问他们:"吃了什么好东西,长得这么结实?"兄弟俩拿出草根给大家瞧。大伙儿都说这东西长得像人的身体,这形如"人身"的根被后人称为"人参"。人参的主要功效有:大补元气,复脉固脱,补脾益肺,生津,安神等。

Ginseng（Ginseng Radix et Rhizoma）

Once upon a time, two brothers in a village of Northeast China, brought with them bows and arrows, furs and dried food to go hunting in the mountains in winter. The next day, it began to snow and went on for three days and nights. The downhill road was blocked by snow. The brothers couldn't go out of the mountains. They found a hollow tree and hided themselves from the wind and snow. In order to save food, they dug up some grass roots to eat around the hole. By accident they dug up some grassy root as thick as a thumb like human limbs. It tasted sweet and they felt more energetic after eating the root. They even got a nosebleed when they ate too much of it. So they ate only little by little each day.

Not until the spring of next year did the brothers return home, full of prey.

The villagers thought that they might have died during the long, cold winter in the mountains. When they saw them back healthy and energetic, they were surprised to ask, "What food have you eaten that made you so strong?" The brothers showed the grass root to everyone. They all said that it looked like a human body. People named it *"ren shen"* (meaning human body). Later it was renamed as ginseng. The main functions of ginseng are: reinforcing *qi*, restoring and nourishing the spleen and the lungs, increasing body fluids and comforting nerves.

小和尚和人参的故事

很久很久以前,山东有个云梦寺,寺里有一老一小两个和尚。老和尚不但无心拜佛,而且天天下山游玩。小和尚在寺中,还时常挨老和尚怪罪刁难,人被折磨得骨瘦如柴。一天,老和尚下山前,给小和尚安排了很多工作。小和尚干活累得腰酸背痛。这时,不知从何处跑来一个穿红肚兜的小孩,不声不响地帮小和尚干起活来。说来也怪,在穿红肚兜小孩的帮助下,活儿很快做完了。此后,只要老和尚下山去,穿红兜肚的小孩就会来帮助小和尚忙这忙那。老和尚返回寺中,小孩就不知去向了。

时间久了,老和尚很奇怪小和尚每次都能把任务完成。就逼迫小和尚说出了实情。老和尚威逼小和尚:"小孩如果再来的时候,你悄悄地把这根穿了红线的针别在他的红肚兜上。"小和尚非常为难,又无法抗拒。终于有一天,红兜肚小孩干完活,准备离开时,小和尚趁其不备将针别在了小孩的肚兜上。第二天,老和尚把小和尚锁在库房中,手持镐头,顺着红线,来到一株老松树下,只见那针插在一棵人参苗上。他高兴极了,举起镐头,恶狠狠地刨下去,不一会就挖出了一个"人参娃"来。

The Story of a Little Monk and Ginseng

Long long ago, there was a Yunmeng Temple in Shandong. Two monks, an old and a young, lived in the temple. The old monk went down the mountain to enjoy life every day rather than worship the Buddha. The young one had to stay in the temple and he was often blamed by the old monk so that he became thin as a bag of bones. One day, before the old monk went down the mountain, he arranged a lot of work for the young one to do which made him so tired that he had a backache. At this time, a child wearing a red bellyband came quietly to help him. With the help of the child, the work was soon finished. After that, as long as the old monk went down the mountain, the little boy would come up to help the young monk. When the old one returned to the temple, the child disappeared.

The old monk felt strange that the little one can finish the task every time. He forced the little monk and threatened, "If the child comes again, pin this needle with a red thread quietly on his red belly pocket." The young monk was very hesitated but could not refuse. One day, the little monk pinned the needle to the little boy's bellyband when he finished his work. The next day, the old monk locked the young in the storehouse. Holding a hoe on his shoulders, the old one came to an old pine tree along the red line. He saw the needle inserted in an old ginseng tree. He was so happy that he raised the hoe and dug it savagely. Soon he dug out a "ginseng boy".

丹 参

丹参是一味常用中药,别名红根、紫丹参、血参根等,这是因其药用的根部呈紫红色之故。此外,民间还有将其称作"丹心"的,这与流传的一个感人故事有关。

相传很久以前,东海岸边的一个渔村里住着一个叫"阿明"的青年。阿明从小丧父,与母亲相依为命,因自幼在风浪中长大,练就了一身好水性,人称"小蛟龙"。有一年,阿明的母亲患了妇科病,经常崩漏下血,请了很多大夫,都未治愈,阿明甚是一筹莫展。正当此时,有人说东海中有个无名岛,岛上生长着一种花开紫蓝色、根呈红色的药草,以这种药草的根煎汤内服,就能治愈其母亲的病。阿明听后,喜出望外,便决定去无名岛采药。

村里的人听说后,都为阿明捏着一把汗,因为去无名岛的海路不但暗礁林立,而且水流湍急,欲上岛者十有九死,犹过"鬼门关"。但病不宜迟,阿明救母心切,毅然决定出海上岛采药。

第二天,阿明就驾船出海了。他凭着高超的水性,绕过了一个个暗礁,冲过了一个个激流险滩,终于闯过"鬼门关"、顺利登上了无名岛。上岸后,他四处寻找那种开着紫蓝色花、根是红色的药草。每找到一棵,便赶快挖出其根,不一会儿就挖了一大捆。返回渔村后,阿明每日按时侍奉母亲服药,母亲的病很快就痊愈了。

村里人对阿明冒死采药为母治病的事,非常敬佩。都说这种药草凝结了阿明的一片丹心,便给这种根红的药草取名"丹心"。后来在流传过程中,取其谐音就变成"丹参"了。

Dan Shen (Salviae Miltiorrhizae Radix et Rhizoma)

Dan Shen is commonly used in traditional Chinese medicine, having the alias as red root, purple Salvia and ginseng root because its roots are purple. In addition, in folklore it was also called *Dan Xin* (meaning "a loyal heart"), which was related to a touching story.

Long long ago, there was a young man named Ah Ming, living in a fishing village at the east coast. His father died when he was young. So he had to live with his mother. Because he was often diving into the sea to fish since childhood, he was good at swimming and was called "little dragon". One day, Ah Ming's mother felt ill of gynecological disease, bleeding from time to time. Doctors could do nothing for her. At that time, some people told him there was an unknown island in East Sea. On the island, there was a herb which has purple-blue flowers and red roots. Taking the root of this herb to boil a decoction and giving it to his mother to drink could cure her illness. On hearing that, Ah Ming was very happy and decided to go to the unknown island to find this herb.

People in the village all worried about him because the sea around the island was so dangerous with many submerged rocks. Yet, his mother's illness could not be delayed, so Ah Ming decided to go. On the second day, Ah Ming sailed to the sea. With his superb swimming skill, he moved round reefs and finally got through "the gates of hell" and boarded on the unknown island. Having got ashore, he began to look for herbs with purple blue flowers and red roots. Each time he found one, he dug out the roots, and soon he gathered a big bundle of them. After returning home, Ah Ming boiled the roots for his mother every day, and his mother recovered quickly.

People in the village admired Ah Ming so much for his fearlessness of death and his loyal heart for his mother. So they named the herb "*Dan Xin*" (a loyal heart). Later, during the spreading, the name was gradually changed to *Dan Shen*.

当　归

相传有个新婚青年要上山采药,对妻子说三年回来,谁知一去,一年无信,二年无音,三年仍不见回来。媳妇因思念丈夫而忧郁悲伤,得了气血亏损的妇女病,后来只好改嫁。谁知后来她的丈夫又回来了。她对丈夫哭诉道:"三年当归你不归,片纸只字也不回,如今我已错嫁人,心如刀割真悔恨。"丈夫也懊悔自己没有按时回来,遂把采集的草药根拿去给媳妇治病,竟然治好了她的妇女病。

从此,人们才知道这种草药根有补血、活血、调经、止痛之效,是一种妇科良药。为汲取"当归不归,娇妻改嫁"的悲剧教训,人们便把它叫作"当归"。

Dang Gui（Angelicae Sinensis Radix）

As the legend has it, there was a newly-married young man who went to the mountains to collect herbs, and promised his wife that he would return in three years. However, he did not come back year after year. And there was not a message from him. His wife was so sorrowful that she caught gynecopathy with *qi* and blood deficiency. Finally, she remarried. One day, to everyone's surprise, the young man came back. She cried and blamed on him, "Why didn't you return on time? Now, I am remarried and sorry for what I had done." The husband felt regretted, too. He used the herb he collected in these three years to treat her and it cured her gynecopathy disease.

Since then, people learned that this herb had the effect of invigorating the circulation of blood, regulating menstruation and relieving pain. It is named *Dang Gui* (meaning "come back on time") in order to remember the tragic lesson of "come back on time or you'll lose your beloved wife".

麝　香

麝香是中国特产的一种名贵药材,以康藏高原及四川阿坝草原为中国麝香的主要产地,销全国,并出口。性温,味辛;入心经、脾经、肝经,有开窍、辟秽、通络、散淤之功能。主治中风、痰厥、惊痫、中恶烦闷、心腹暴痛、跌打损伤、痈疽肿毒。孕妇忌用。关于麝香,流传着这样一个故事。

从前,一对唐姓父子居住在深山里,以打猎为生。一天,父子俩在深山老林打猎,儿子为追捕一只野雉,不慎掉下山涧。儿子虽倒在洞里动弹不得,却贪婪地吸着山涧飘来的缕缕奇香。这奇特的香气,沁人心脾,伤痛好像逐渐消散。唐老汉扒开泥土发现一个鸡蛋大小、长着细毛的香囊。不久儿子的伤不治而愈。

后来,每遇到穷人跌打损伤,唐老汉就用香囊为其治疗。此事被县太爷得知,便派衙役将香囊抢去,交给小妾收藏。小妾将香囊随身携带,哪知已怀孕三月的胎儿坠了下来。唐老汉失去香囊后,上山打猎时便加倍留意。他终于发现,雄性麝的腹部有一装着分泌物的囊袋,这个囊袋就叫"麝香"。

She Xiang (Moschus)

Musk is a kind of rare medicinal herb in China, produced originally in the Tibetan Plateau and the Aba grassland in Sichuan. It is a best seller at home and abroad. Warm and spicy, it works for heart, spleen and liver meridian, having the effects of inducing resuscitation, monarch shouts, dredging, and dissipating blood stasis. It can treat stroke, phlegm reversal, epilepsy, depression, evil henchmen sudden pain, bruises, carbuncle swollen poison. Pregnant women are prohibited to use it. As for musk, there is such a story.

Once upon a time, a father named Tang and his son were hunting in the mountains. One day, when they were chasing a pheasant, the son accidentally fell off into a hole. Unable to move in the hole, he greedily inhaled the floating wisps of a strange fragrance. This peculiar sweet smell gladdened his heart and refreshed his mind, making his pain fade away. The old man, Tang, wiped out the dirt and found an egg-sized sachet with long hairs. After inhaling the fragrance of the sachet, it was not long before the injury of his son healed.

Later, Tang treated many people who have traumatic injuries with this sachet. Knowing of the anecdote, the county magistrate sent a panel to grab away that sachet and gave it to his young concubine as a token. The young woman brought it with her wherever she went, only to find that her three-month pregnancy had been aborted. The old man, Tang, was watchful to find another sachet when he hunted in the mountains after losing the first one. At last, he found that it was a bag filled with secretions which was attached to the abdomen of a male deer. That is "musk".

山 药

关于山药的来历,有一个美丽的传说:古时候,焦作一带有一个小国,叫野王国(今沁阳市)。由于国小势弱,常被一些大国欺负。一年冬天,一个大国派军队入侵野王国,野王国的将士们虽然拼死奋战,但最终因军力不足战败了。战败的军队逃进了深山,偏又遇到天降大雪,大国的军队封锁了所有的出山道路,欲将野王国的军队困死山中。大雪纷飞,将士们饥寒交迫,许多人已经奄奄一息。正当绝望之际,有人发现一种植物的根茎,吃起来味道还不错,而且这种植物漫山遍野都是。士兵们喜出望外,纷纷挖这种植物的根茎吃。更为神奇的是,吃了这种根茎后,将士们体力大增,就连吃了这种植物的藤蔓和叶枝的马也变得强壮无比。士气大振的野王国军队终于夺回了失地,保住了国家。后来,将士们为纪念这种植物,给它取名"山遇"。随着更多人食用这种植物,人们发现它还具有治病健身的效果,遂将"山遇"改名为"山药"。

山药有补脾养胃、生津益肺、补肾涩精的功效,应用于脾虚食少,久泻不止,白带过多,肺虚久咳,肾虚遗精,带下,尿频,虚热消渴等病症。

Shan Yao (Dioscoreae Rhizoma)

There is a beautiful legend about the origin of yam. In ancient times, there was a small country named Ye Wang Guo (now Qinyang, Henan Province). It was a weak state, often bullied by some big countries. One winter, a large country sent troops to invade Ye Wang Guo. Although the soldiers fought desperately, they were defeated eventually. The defeated army retreated into the mountains, but encountered heavy snow. The armies of the great powers sealed off all the roads, trying to trap the army of Ye Wang Guo. It was snowing in great flakes, the soldiers were cold and hungry, and many were dying. In desperation, some soldiers dug the root of a plant, which tasted good and was all over the hill. The soldiers were overjoyed to dig out the roots. Even more miraculously, after eating this root, the soldiers' strength increased, and even the horses that ate the vines and branches of this plant became stronger. The morale of the army was greatly boosted and they finally recaptured the lost land and saved the country. Later, in honor of this plant, the soldiers named it "*Shan Yu*" (meaning "meeting by chance in the mountains"). More people ate the plants and found that it had the effect of treating disease and keeping fitness, hence "*Shan Yu*" was renamed "*Shan Yao*" (meaning "a herb in the mountains").

Shan Yao has the effects of nourishing spleen and stomach, and monishing lungs and kidney. It's applied to the spleen deficiency, lung deficiency, cough, kidney deficiency, urinary frequency, and deficiency of heat and thirst.

枸杞子

宋朝时期,传说某日有位在朝使者奉命离京赴银川办事,在途中见一位娇柔婀娜、满头青丝、年约十六七岁的姑娘手执竹竿,口里嘀咕唠叨着在追打一个白发苍苍、弓腰驼背的八九十岁老头。老头前躲后藏很是可怜,使者见状便下马挡住那姑娘责问:"此老者是你何人,你应尊敬老人,为何如此对待他?"那姑娘回答:"这人是我的曾孙儿。"使者惊道:"那你为何要打他呢?"答曰:"家有良药他不肯服食,年纪轻轻就这样老态龙钟的,头发也白了,牙齿也掉光了,就因为这个。所以我才要教训他。"使者好奇地问道:"你今年多少岁了?"姑娘应声说:"我今年已有372岁了!"使者听后更加惊异,忙问:"你是用什么方法得到高寿的呢?"姑娘说:"我没有什么神秘方法,只是常年服用了一种叫枸杞子的药,据说可以使人与天地齐寿。"使者听罢,急忙记录了下来。被称为"神仙药"的枸杞子有滋补肝肾,益精明目之效,用于治疗虚劳精亏、腰膝酸痛、眩晕耳鸣、内热消渴、血虚萎黄、目昏不明等病症。

Goji (Lycii Fructus)

In the Song Dynasty (960 – 1279), it was said that one day an emissary from the capital city went to Yinchuan on business. On the way he met a graceful young girl, who seemed to be sixteen or seventeen years old with black hair. The girl, holding a bamboo stick, nagged and chased a grey-haired and crookbacked old man who was about 80 or 90 years old. It was a pitiful scene to see an old man running for a shelter. On seeing that, the emissary immediately came down from his horse and asked the girl, "Who is the old man? You should respect the elderly. Why do you treat him like that?" The girl replied, "He is my great-grandson." The emissary was shocked, "Why did you beat him?" The girl said, "There was an effective medicine in the house and he refused to take it. So, he looks old and clumsy at a young age. His hair is white and the teeth are gone. That's why I'm going to beat him." The emissary was even more curiously, asking, "How old are you?" The girl replied, "I'm 372 years old." The emissary was greatly surprised, and asked hastily, "What secret do you have to keep longevity?" The girl said, "I don't have any mysterious methods. I just took a herb called Goji all the year round. It is said that it can make people live as long as heaven and earth." Having heard of that, the emissary recorded it quickly and called it "immortal fairy medlar". Goji has functions of nourishing kidney, enriching essence and improving eyesight. It is used to treat consumptive sperm loss, waist and knee pains, dizziness and tinnitus, heat diabetes, blood deficiency chlorosis, unknown dizziness and blurred vision.

八珍汤

傅山是我国一代名医,他医德高尚、医术精湛,以关心百姓疾苦,提高百姓身心健康水平为己任。在中医药理学与营养学理论的指导下,他研制出了药膳养生食品"八珍汤"。"八珍汤"是由八种中草药组成,经过精细复杂的工艺制作而成的一种糊状食品,经常食用可达到舒筋活血、养心益肾、补血生阳、健脾和胃的效用。

"八珍汤"制作时选料讲究、程序复杂,方法技巧要求十分严格。在选料备料时,要做到备料全、选料精的要求。精选肥嫩上等羊肉做原料,经过清洗、净肉、加辅料煮炖、出锅晾存等诸道工序将肉煮熟,并将羊汤、羊油撇出备用;同时将诸种辅料严格按照既定制法或煨、或腌、或煮、或蒸,做好备用。制作"八珍汤"就是将上述材料按照既定的程序、比例,上火熬煮,并加入黄酒调制而成。

Ba Zhen Soup

Fu Shan, a famous doctor in ancient China, had noble medical ethics and high medical skills. He regarded the concern of people and the improvement of people's health as his own responsibility. Under the guidance of the theory of traditional Chinese medicine and Dietetics, he manufactured through refined and complicated process, the famous "Ba Zhen Soup", which consists of eight kinds of Chinese herbal medicine, having the effect of relaxing the sinews, invigorating the circulation of blood, nourishing the heart, benefiting the kidney, enriching the blood, generating yang, strengthening spleen, and normalizing stomach.

To cook Ba Zhen Soup, the selection of materials is very strict and the process is complex. To select and prepare the materials, it is required that the materials are all ready and cream. Fat and tender superior mutton is carefully chosen as a raw material. The mutton is cooked through these processes: cleaning meat, removing bones and skins, adding accessories to stew, fishing the meat out of the pot, drying the meat out and preserving it for use. Then the mutton soup and mutton tallow are skimmed. At the same time, all kinds of accessories are strictly prepared in accordance with the established method to simmer, pickle, boil or steam. Briefly speaking, the process of doing it is that the above materials are strictly boiled in accordance with the established procedure and proportion. Ultimately, rice wine is added to the soup to modulate its flavor.

熟地治瘟疫

在唐朝时,有一年,黄河中下游发生瘟疫,流行很广,很多老百姓失去了生命,县太爷来到神农山的药王庙祈求老天保佑。这时,从庙的外边来了一个人,他送给县太爷一株根状的草药,送药人将这个药草称为"地皇",意思是皇天赐药,并告诉他神农山北边的洼地里有许多这种药草。县太爷非常高兴,立即安排了很多人上山采挖,老百姓吃了这个药草的汁疾病就痊愈了,百姓们得救了。瘟疫过后,百姓们把它引种到自家农田里种植,并且流传到全国各地。因为它的颜色发黄,百姓便把"地皇"叫成"地黄"了。

Shudi (Rehmanniae Radix Praeparata) Treated Plague

In the Tang Dynasty (618-907), one year a plague occurred in the middle and lower reaches of the Yellow River. The epidemic was widespread and many people lost their lives. The county magistrate came to the Yaowang Temple in Shennong Mountain to pray for God's blessing. At this moment, a man came from outside of the temple. He gave the magistrate a root-shaped herb. The medicine-giver called the herb "*dihuang*", meaning it is given by heaven, and told him that there were many such herbs in the marsh north of Shennong Mountain. The county magistrate was so happy that he arranged a trip to the mountain to dig this herb immediately. The epidemic was stopped and the people were saved by taking the juice of this herb. After the plague, the herb was replanted in people's farmlands all over the country. Because of its yellow color, people called it "*dihuang*" (yellow farmland).

黄 精

古时有一肺痨患者,自知将不久于人世,就跑到深山躲了起来。几年后,他非但没死,身体反而强壮起来,说话声如洪钟。一日,华佗行医路过此处,听了此事就决心弄个明白。于是,他找到了这位"神仙"。从这位"神仙"口中得知,他是长期食用一种开绿花、长黄根的植物治好了病。华佗顺口说道:"真乃药中之精啊!"于是就有了"黄精"之名,并一直流传至今。

黄精属于百合科植物,用于阴虚肺燥,干咳少痰,以及肺肾阴虚的劳嗽、久咳等,对延缓衰老,改善脾、肾功能不足有一定的疗效。

Huang Jing (Polygonati Rhizoma)

In ancient times, there was a man who suffered from tuberculosis. He thought that he would die soon. Therefore he hid himself in the mountains. A few years later, not only didn't he die, he was physically strong and his voice sounded like a brass bell. One day when Hua Tuo passed by and learned about the story during his practice of medicine, he decided to figure out the truth of this story. Therefore, Hua Tuo found him and learned the secret. This guy happened to consume a kind of herb with green flowers and yellow roots, in the end his disease was cured. Then Hua Tuo said unwittingly, "It is really the essence of medicine!" So the herb got the name "the yellow essence" (*Huang Jing*), which had been passing down till now.

Huang Jing belongs to the liliaceous family. It can be used for *yin* deficiency and phlegm-heat, cough with little phlegm, labor cough that caused by thirst of lung and kidney. And it also has a certain curative effect on anti-aging and improving spleen and kidney deficiency.

何首乌

何首乌具有补血,黑须发,久服长筋骨,益精髓,益寿延年的功效。现代药理学也证明其具有降低血脂、血糖的作用,可以预防冠心病、脑动脉硬化等疾病。它的原名叫交藤,因为何首乌经常服用这个药,于是就将它称作何首乌。

何首乌是顺州南河县人,祖父叫能嗣,父名叫延秀。能嗣本来的名字叫田儿,生来就虚弱多病,年已五十八岁,尚无妻室儿女,经常羡慕道家方术,随同老师入山中修道。一天喝醉了酒睡在山野之中,忽然看见有蔓藤二株,相距三尺多远,苗蔓相缠,良久才分开,如此缠绕相交。田儿看了异常惊奇,到天明即挖去此藤的根回家,问之于人,皆不认识。后来有一位山中老人忽然来到,看后说:"你既然无嗣育,这藤如此异常,恐怕是神仙之药,为何不把它服下去?"于是就把藤捣碎为沫,空腹用酒冲服一钱,过了数月后,自觉身体康壮。因此常常服这药。后又将药量加至二钱。过了一年后,不仅原来身上的疾病痊愈了,头发也多变黑了,面容也年轻了许多。十年之内,就生了几个男孩,于是田儿就改名叫"能嗣"。又把这个药给其子延秀吃,结果他们都活到了一百六十岁。延秀生首乌,首乌服此药,也生了几个儿子,活到一百三十岁,头发仍然乌黑。有个叫李安期的人,与首乌同为邻居,相处也很亲近,他获得此方,其寿命也延长了许多,遂将此事记载而传了下来。

He Shouwu (Polygoni Multiflori Radix)

He Shouwu is medicated to nourish blood, strengthen bones, make hair black, enrich the essence and prolong life. Modern pharmacology also proves that it has the effect of reducing fat in the blood and blood sugar, and can prevent diseases such as coronary heart disease and cerebral arteriosclerosis. Polygonum multiflorum was originally called *Jiaoteng* and later called *He Shouwu*, because a person named He Shouwu often ate it. Latter people called it after him.

He Shouwu lived in Nanhe County of Shunzhou. His grandfather was named Nengsi (meaning "able to produce offspring"), and his father's name was Yanxiu. Nengsi was originally named Tian'er, and had been weak since childhood. When he was fifty-eight years old, he still had no wife nor children. He admired the Daoist approach to immortality, and often went deep into the mountains to learn the Daoist way with some teachers. One day he was drunk and slept in the mountains. Suddenly he awoke and saw two intertwining vines. He was surprised and curious, so he dug out the root of the vine the next morning and took it home. He consulted others about the vine but nobody knew about it. Later an old man suddenly came and said, "Since you have no children and encountered this plant by accident, maybe it is a medicine from heaven. Why not take this extraordinary herb?" So he crashed the herb into powder, taking it with wine into the empty stomach. A few months later, he felt strong and robust. Since then he often took the drug and later increased the dosage. A year later, he recovered from physical weakness with growing black hair, and his face looked young. He had several sons within ten years, and thus changed his name into Nengsi. Later he asked his sons to take this drug. They all lived to 160 years old. Yanxiu has a son named Shouwu, who also had several sons, and they all lived to 130 years old while their hair was still black. There was a man named Li Anqi, who was one of Shouwu's neighbors and got along well with Shouwu, and he got the prescription and extended his longevity. It is he who recorded the story.

橘井泉香

葛洪《神仙传·苏仙公传》记载:苏耽在汉文帝的时候(公元前180年—公元前157年)受天命为天仙,天上的仪仗队降落苏宅迎接苏耽。苏耽在辞别母亲、超脱凡俗时告知母亲:"明年天下将流行瘟疫,咱们家庭院中的井水和橘树能治疗瘟疫。患瘟疫的人,给他井水一升,橘叶一枚,吃下橘叶、喝下井水就能治愈了。"后来果然像他所说的那样,前来求取井水、橘叶的人很多,都被治愈了。于是医学史上就有了"橘井泉香"的典故。

Well Water and Tangerine Leaves

Ge Hong recorded a story about the biography of Su Xiangong in the book *Fairy Biographies*. During the Han Dynasty(180 B.C.–157 B.C.), a filial man named Su Dan was appointed as a celestial being. One day, the guard of honor from the welkin landed in Su's home to welcome him to heaven. When Su left, he said to his mother,"Next year, a plague will break out here. Well water and tangerine leaves in our courtyard could treat the disease. Give those who suffer from the plague a liter of water and an orange leaf. After eating them, the patient could be cured." As he predicted, the nasty disease broke out in the following year. As he said, people came to his house to ask for the water and leaves and they were all rescued. Thus, the story of well water and tangerine leaves was recorded in the history of Chinese medicine.

葛根的传说

相传在唐朝的时候(618—907年),有座山,山脚下住着一对夫妻,男的读书,希望考取功名,女的耕种,供养家庭。十年寒窗苦读,丈夫高中进士,本是喜从天降,但是丈夫却烦恼满怀,只因长安城里富家女子个个都很漂亮,丰盈美丽,想到自己家里妻子长年劳作,瘦弱不堪,于是有心休妻。他托乡人带信回家,妻子打开只见两句诗"缘似落花如流水,驿道春风是牡丹",妻子明白丈夫看不上自己了,将要把自己抛弃,终日茶饭不思,以泪洗面,更是容颜憔悴。

山神得知后,怜爱善良苦命的女子,梦中指引这位妻子每日上山挖食葛根,不久,此女竟脱胎换骨,变得丰盈美丽,光彩照人。但丈夫托走乡人后,思来想去:患难之妻,怎能抛弃! 于是快马加鞭,赶回故里,发现妻子变得异常美丽,更加大喜过望,夫妻团圆,共同过上了美好的生活。

The Legend of Gegen (Puerariae Lobatae Radix)

As legend has it that in the Tang Dynasty (618 – 907), there was a mountain, where a couple lived at its foot. The husband hoped to get fame by taking the official service exams while the wife was engaged in farming to support the family. After ten years of hard study, the husband succeeded in the imperial examinations. This was a good thing but the husband met with a trouble because he felt the temptation was great for rich ladies in the capital city were so beautiful and slender. Thinking that his wife was thin and weak for years' hard labor, he decided to divorce his wife. So he asked a villager to take a letter home. His wife opened it and saw two lines of poetry: The fate is like the falling flowers and flowing water while spring breeze is just like the peony on the post road. The wife understood that her husband looked down upon her and wanted to abandon her. She spent all day crying without eating or drinking which made her haggard.

When the god of the mountain learned this, he took pity on the kind-hearted and miserable woman. The god led the wife to go up to the mountain every day to dig and eat kudzu roots in her dream. The woman was completely reborn and became slender and beautiful. After the husband gave the letter to the fellow villager, he thought to himself: How can a wife in distress be abandoned! So he rode back home quickly. Finding his wife became unusually beautiful, he was more than happy and then they had a better life together.

麻沸散的发明

华佗在鲁南地区(今山东省)为一个胳膊上生了毒疮的小孩动手术。那孩子连蹦带跳,疼得死去活来。这件事深深触痛了华佗的心。他想:"要是制成一种药,先让病人服下,然后动手术时既不痛苦,又能治好病,那该多好!"

有一天,几个小伙子抬来一个昏迷不醒的汉子,求华佗医治。华佗问:"这人伤在哪里?""他和人打架,让人打断了肋骨!"一个小伙子忙说。华佗给伤者解开衣服一看,左胸下血肉模糊,肋骨都露出来了。他让小伙子们按住伤者,然后忙用药水擦洗伤口,开始动手术。这时,华佗才发现,整个手术过程中,那人不仅没有挣扎,连一声呻吟都没发出。忽然,一股酒气扑鼻而来。一问,原来那伤者喝得酩酊大醉,这时还酣睡在梦中呢。这一例手术给华佗极大启发。只要制成一种药让病人服下后能像喝醉酒一样睡着,手术就顺利得多了。

华佗开始研究麻醉剂。经过一次次的试验、改进,一种用浓酒配制的中药麻醉剂——麻沸散制成。麻沸散有麻醉作用,能减轻病人因手术带来的痛苦,它的发明为中医药发展作出了巨大贡献。

The Invention of Anesthesia Powder

When Hua Tuo was operating in the southern area of Lu (now Shandong Province) on a child's arm where a carbuncle lay, the child felt so painful that he twisted and turned. This case deeply touched the heart of Hua Tuo. He thought, "If I could produce a medicine to make the patient feel no pain during the surgery, that would be wonderful!"

One day, some guys brought an unconscious man to Hua Tuo for operation.

Hua Tuo asked: "What's wrong with him?" One of the guys replied: "He had a fight and broke his ribs." Then Hua Tuo examined the man and found that his left chest was covered by blood and broken ribs were exposed out. He asked the boys to put down the wounded, and then scrubbed the wound with medicine to begin the surgery. To his surprise, Hua Tuo found that the wounded did not utter a single groan during the operation. Suddenly, he smelt the fumes of wine and knew that the wounded was drunk. It is a great inspiration to Hua Tuo! So long as he could find the drug to make the patients sleep in surgery like being drunk, the surgery would be much smoother.

Then Hua Tuo began to study anesthetics. A mixture of Chinese liquor anesthesia powder, which can reduce the patients' pain during surgery, was made after repeated tests and improvements. The invention of anesthesia powder has greatly contributed to the development of Chinese medicine.

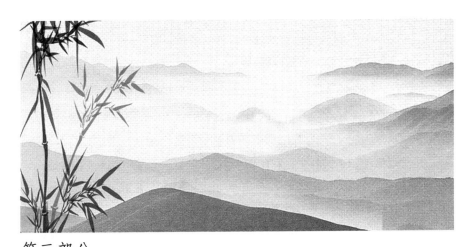

第三部分

Part Three

成语与俗语

Idioms and Proverbs

不可救药

西周(公元前 1046—公元前 771 年)的厉王,生活奢侈,骄奢淫逸,残酷地压迫和剥削人民。当时有位忠臣叫凡伯,常冒死劝谏,但厉王根本不听。那些厉王宠信的奸臣们都嘲笑凡伯。凡伯眼看着国势日衰,内心十分焦急,于是写了一首诗警告这帮人。大意如下:不是我老了,才说这些话,忧患没到来时还可防止;假若忧患越积越多,就像燃旺了的火焰,就没法救了。果然,不久以后老百姓终于忍无可忍,冲进王宫,把周厉王赶到很远的地方去了。周厉王在那儿待了十四年,直到死去。

"不可救药"形容病重到不能用药救活,后比喻事物坏到无法挽救的地步。

Beyond Remedy

In the Western Zhou Dynasty (1046 B. C. – 771 B. C.) , luxurious and dissipated King Li oppressed and exploited the people cruelly. At that time, Fan Bo, a loyal minister, often tried to remonstrate, but the King turned a deaf ear to him and those treacherous court officials all laughed at him. Seeing the decline of the country with worry, Fan wrote a poem to warn those people as follows: Worry could be prevented when it does not come. Accumulating troubles are like flaming fire, there's no way for us to put it out. As he predicted, before long the civilians could not bear any more and rushed into the Palace. King Li was deported far away and stayed there for fourteen years until death.

The phrase "beyond remedy" indicates that the disease is too serious to be cured, and later the metaphor means that something is too bad to be saved.

折　肱

折肱,喻指良医。《左传·定公三十年》曰:"三折肱知为良医。"《楚辞·九章》曰:"九折臂而成医兮,吾至今乃知其信然。"朱熹集注:"人九折臂,更历方药,乃成良医,故吾于今,乃知作忠造怨之语,为诚然也。《左传》曰:三折肱为良医。亦此意也。"后遂以"三折肱""九折臂"以喻良医。以此命名者,如明代吴承昊(1368—1644年)《折肱漫录》。

Zhe Gong（Humerus）

"Zhe Gong"（meaning "broken arms"）refers to a good doctor. According to *Zuo Zhuan · 30 years of Ding Gong*, "Having been broken in your arms for three times, you will understand how to be a good doctor." *Chu Ci · Nine Chapters* also has this saying, "After the arm was broken for nine times, you will become a good doctor. I believe it a truth." Notes from *Zhu Xi*: When a person's arm was broken nine times and experienced various kinds of treatment, he will become a good doctor in the end. I know it's correct, not the resentment. *Zuo Zhuan* also has this saying, "People whose arm was broken for three times must know the method to cure it." Later, people always use the words "San Zhe Gong" and "Jiu Zhe Bi" as metaphors to describe a good doctor. For instance, Wu Chenghao（1368 – 1644）of the Ming Dynasty wrote the book *A Record of Zhe Gong*.

病入膏肓

晋景公病重,打算去秦国聘请医术高明的人来给自己治病。秦桓公派了一个名叫缓的秦国医生来给他医治。医生还没到来之前,晋景公做了一个梦,梦见疾病变成了两个童子在自己的身体里谈话。一个说:"晋景公这回请的人,医术十分高明。那个医生来了,会用药伤害我们。这回怎么逃啊?"另一个说:"我们躲在肓之上,膏之下,那是药力达不到的地方,能拿我们怎么办?"

医生到了,说:"病无法治疗。在肓的上面,膏的下面,用热水焐也不行,是针灸的力量也达不到的。药无法治,病不能治疗。"晋景公听后说:"这是良医呀!"晋景公赠予他厚礼然后送他回去了。

Sick to the Vitals

Duke Jing of the State of Jin(266-420) was ill. He sent an official to the State of Qin to find good doctors. The duke of Qin, Huangong, then sent a physician named Huan to see what could be done for him. Before Huan's arrival, Duke Jing dreamed that his disease had become two kids chatting in his body. One of them said, "The coming physician is very competent. I'm afraid he will hurt us. Let's run away." The other replied, "No. We'll stay somewhere above *huang* and below *gao*. He can do nothing to us".

The physician came. After the diagnosis, he concluded, "There's no cure for the disease. It lies above *huang* and below *gao*, where no moxibustion can be applied nor acupuncture be manipulated, and drugs will never reach there. Nothing can be done for it." Hearing these words, Duke Jin commended Huan as a truly competent doctor and sent him home with great rewards.

Note: In traditional Chinese medicine, *Gao* means fat, *huang* means pericardium, and *gaohuang* refers to the place in the body that the medicine cannot reach. Gao huang(BL43) is also an acupoint on people's back.

大葫芦

　　一天,惠子见到庄子,讲了这样一件事:"惠王赐给我大葫芦的种子,我把它种在地里。不久,真的结了个很大的葫芦,恐怕装得下五石谷子。我也是第一次看到这么大的葫芦,高兴极了。但它却解决不了我一点儿实际问题。一气之下,我把它砸碎了。"庄子听了,十分惋惜地说:"您这样轻易地把这么好的葫芦打碎了,实在是太可惜了。"

　　惠子不等庄子把话说完,抢着问道:"您觉得可惜,您想用它做什么呢?"庄子心平气和地给惠子讲了一个故事:宋国有一个人,会制作防止冻疮的药。他家祖祖辈辈靠给人漂洗棉絮为生。有人听说后就登门拜访。愿出百斤黄金买他家的祖传秘方。全家一道商量这件事后说:"我看还是卖给他吧!咱们世世代代为人漂洗,收入少得可怜。现在如果能卖掉药方,一下子就能得到一大笔钱。不能错过这个机会啊!"于是,全家同意卖掉秘方。

　　庄子接着说:"那个人得了秘方,像得了千金宝贝。就去游说吴王。这时,越国侵犯吴国。吴王便派他去带兵迎战。当时,正是冬天,天气十分寒冷。越、吴两军在水上交战。吴军因为有了这个秘方,全军上下没有一个人手脚冻裂。最后大破越军。为此,吴王大大奖赏了那个人,封他做了大官。

　　"能防止手足冻裂的冻疮药,有的人用它来封官进爵。有的人则只能用来为人漂洗棉絮。这是为什么? 这是因为有人小材大用,有人却大材小用的缘故。"说到这儿,庄子停了下来,想了想又接着说:"先生,您也应该学会利用大葫芦呀! 我以为用作瓢舀水,倒不如把它用作舟楫渡江河湖海。不是比现在更好吗?"惠子听了连连点头,承认庄子比自己高明。他感叹说:"看来,我还是个心眼不开窍的人呀!"

The Big Gourd

One day, Hui Zi(390 B.C.-317 B.C.) met Zhuang Zi(369 B.C.-286 B. C.) and told him this story, "King Hui bestowed upon me some big gourd seeds, which I planted in the earth. Soon afterwards a big gourd which could hold 5 *dan* of rice really grew in the field. Never before have I seen such a big gourd, so I was very pleased. But it couldn't solve any of my practical problems. I was so disappointed that I smashed it." When Zhuang Zi heard of this, he felt very sorry and said, "It's really a pity that you smashed such a good gourd so rashly."

Hui Zi couldn't wait for Zhuang Zi to finish his words and asked, "You feel it a pity, then what would you use it for?" Zhuang Zi told Hui Zi a story calmly. There was a man in the State of Song, who could make medicine for preventing chilblains. For generations his family made a living by bleaching and washing cotton wadding for others. Someone heard of this and visited their house. He was willing to pay 100 catties of gold to buy the secret prescription. The whole family discussed about the matter. The man said, "I think we had better sell it to him. We have bleached and washed for others for generations with a pitiful income. If we sell the prescription now, we can get a large sum of money at once. We shouldn't miss this opportunity!" Consequently, the whole family agreed to sell the secret prescription.

Zhuang Zi continued, "The man who got the prescription felt as if he had gotten 1,000 pieces of gold. He went to the King of Wu to sell this description. At that time, the State of Yue invaded Wu. The King of Wu sent the man to lead his troops to battle. It was winter then, and the weather was very cold. The armies of the two States fought in water. As the Wu army had this secret prescription, not a single soldier in the army suffered from frostbite of hands or feet. In the end, they defeated the Yue army. For this, the King of Wu rewarded that man generously and offered him a high post. "

"Some people use the medicine for preventing chilblains to get high posts and titles, while others only use it to bleach and wash cotton wadding for a small income. Why? This is because some people can put inferior timber to big use whereas others put fine timber only to petty use." Zhuang Zi stopped at this point, thought for a while, and then continued again, "Sir, you should also learn to utilize your large gourd. I think, instead of using the gourd as a ladle for water, it would be better to use it as a floating boat to cross rivers and lakes. Won't it be better than the present state?" After hearing this, Hui Zi nodded repeatedly and admitted that Zhuang Zi was wiser than him. He said with a sigh, "It seems that I am a person with a muddled head after all."

讳疾忌医

一次,古代名医扁鹊到了齐国。齐国国君田午热情地招待他。扁鹊见到田午,认真地对他说:"目前,您的肌表部位有疾病,要是不治,会发展蔓延下去。"

田午是个很自信的人,他听后不以为然地说:"我没有病"。待扁鹊退下后,他便对旁人说:"医生就是喜欢靠治疗没有病的人来炫耀自己的本领。我才不信呢!"

过了五天,扁鹊去见田午,说:"您的病现在到了血脉,不治恐怕要加重了!"田午说:"我没有病!"脸上显露出厌烦和不高兴的神色。

又过了五天。扁鹊再一次向田午提出忠告:"您的病现已深入到肠胃,再不治疗就不可收拾了!"这次,田午竟拂袖而去。

再过了五天,扁鹊碰见田午,转身便走。田午感到纳闷,派人追上去询问其中的缘故。扁鹊回答说:"当初,国君的病仅在肌表,汤药和灸法可以治;在血脉,针刺可以治;在肠胃,药酒尚可治,现在病入骨髓,即便是神仙下凡也没法医治,我更不敢主动请求医治了。"

五天后,田午果然感到浑身不舒服,病情很快加重,这时他想起扁鹊,连忙派人去找,然而扁鹊已经借故离去。没过几日,田午便死了。

这个成语故事告诉我们:有了疾病,应该积极治疗,若讳疾忌医,到头来只会害自己。对待工作、学习中的缺点和错误也一样,应该及时发现,及时纠正。

Refuse to Be Treated for Fear That Others Will Know About the Illness

Once upon a time, Bian Que(407 B.C.–310 B.C.), a famous doctor in ancient China, arrived in the state of Qi. Tian Wu, the King of Qi (1,044 B.C. -221 B.C.), welcomed him with hospitality. Looking at Tian seriously, Bian said, "There is a disease in the surface of your skin. If you do not treat it right away, it will be getting worse."

Tian was a confident man. He didn't care about what Bian said, so he told Bian that he wasn't sick. After Bian's leaving, he talked to others, "Doctors like to show their skills by treating people with no disease. I don't believe what he said!"

Five days later, Bian met Tian again and reminded him that his illness had got into his blood, and it would get worse without treatment. But Tian had a firm faith in his health, he showed boredom and displeasure on his face.

Another five days passed, Bian admonished Tian of his illness again, "Your disease has been deep into the stomach and intestines now. If you don't treat it, there will be no cure anymore!" Tian was angry and turned away.

Five days later, Bian came across Tian, but he turned around and walked away. Tian was puzzled and sent someone to inquire about the reason. Bian said, "At the very start, the disease is only on the surface, and it can be treated with a herbal and moxibustion therapy. In blood, it could be healed by acupuncture. In intestines and stomach, it can be cured with medicinal liquor. But now the disease has entered the bone marrow, no one can save him even the God, how can I ask for giving a medical treatment!"

Another five days later, Tian felt uncomfortable, as the illness became worse and worse. He sent servants to look for Bian, but Bian had left Qi. Several days later, Tian died.

From the story we know that if you have a disease, you should treat it immediately. If you refuse to be treated for fear that others will know about your illness, you will be hurt in the end. The same is true of your shortcomings and mistakes in work and study, which should be discovered and corrected promptly.

起死回生

有一次,扁鹊路过虢国,看见全国上下都在举行祈祷,一打听,方知是虢太子死了。太子的侍从告诉他,虢太子清晨突然死去。

扁鹊问:"已经掩埋了吗?"

侍从回答说:"还没有。他死了还不过半日哩!"

扁鹊请求进去看看,并说虢太子也许还有生还的希望。

侍从睁大了眼睛,怀疑地说:"先生,你在跟我开玩笑吧!我只听说上古时候的名医俞跗有起死回生的本领。若你能像他那样倒差不多。要不然,连小孩儿也不会相信的。"

扁鹊见侍从不信任自己,很是着急,须知救人要紧哪。他灵机一动,说:"你要是不相信我的话,那么,你去看看太子,他的鼻翼一定还在扇动,他的大腿内侧一定还是温暖的。"

侍从半信半疑地将话告诉了国王。国王十分诧异,忙把扁鹊迎进宫中,痛哭流涕地说:"久闻你医术高明,今日有幸相助。拜托你看看我儿子吧。"

扁鹊一面安慰国王,一面让弟子磨制石针,针刺太子头顶的百会穴。一会儿,太子渐渐苏醒过来,扁鹊又让弟子用药物灸病人的两胁,太子便能慢慢地坐起来。经过中药的进一步调理,二十来天后就康复如初了。

这事很快传遍各地,扁鹊走到哪里,哪里就有人说:"他就是使死人复活的医生!"扁鹊听了,谦逊地笑着说:"我哪里能使死人生还呢,太子患的是'尸厥'证,本来就没有死,我只不过是使他苏醒过来罢了。"

以后,人们常用"起死回生"这个词来形容医生的高超技艺。有些病家有时为了感谢医生,送上一块"扁鹊再世"的横匾,也是颂扬医生医技高超的意思。

Make the Dead Come back to Life

Bian Que was a famous doctor in the Spring and Autumn Period. Once, he passed by the country of Guo and saw that people in the whole country were moaning for someone. He asked the passer-by and was told that the king's son had suddenly died in the morning.

Bian Que asked, "Has he been buried?"

The Prince's attendant replied, "Not yet, he died just half a day ago."

Bian Que thought maybe the prince was still alive and wanted to have a look.

The attendant eyed him and said doubtedly, "Sir, are you kidding me? So far as I know, only the famous doctor, Yu Fu, in ancient times, had the ability to bring the dying back to life. Unless you have the same skill, otherwise, even kids wouldn't believe you."

Seeing that the attendant didn't believe him, but it is urgent to save a life, suddenly he came up with an idea and said, "If you don't trust me, you may go back to see the prince. His nostrils were still stirring, and his inner thighs are warm."

The attendant told the king dubiously. The king was so surprised that he invited Bian Que into the Palace and said to him with tears, "It has been a long time since I heard of your high medical skills. It's my fortune to meet you in my country. Please save my son."

Bian Que comforted the king, and asked his student to grind a stone needle. And then he needled Baihui acupoint on the top of the prince's head. In an instance, the prince gradually woke up. Bian Que told the student to do moxibustion on the prince's *Liangxie* accupoints. Soon the prince could sit up slowly. After the further treatment of traditional Chinese medicine, the prince got recovered in about 20 days.

This story spread all over the country in no time. Wherever Bian Que went, people pointed to hime and said, "He is the doctor who brought the dying back to life!" Bian Que replied, with a modest smile, "I can't do that. The prince was suffering from the 'fake death' (syncope). He wasn't really dead, and I only called him up."

Since then people often use "to make the dead come back to life" to praise a doctor's high skills. People would even give a plague "Rebirth of Bian Que" to a doctor for praising his superb medical skills.

洞见症结

扁鹊,战国人,是我国古代一位十分著名的医生,他的医术高明,救死扶伤,无论在史书中还是民间传说中都有许多关于他的故事。但是他年轻的时候并不是一个医生,而是在一家旅店中做事,在这样的环境中他可以接触到许多从事各行各业的人,后来他认识了一个叫做长桑君的民间医生。长桑君的医术很好,又常住在扁鹊所在的那家旅店,于是扁鹊就经常向他求教。

在那个时代,无论是什么技艺都是父子相传而不传外人的,医术当然也不例外。可是长桑君孤身一人,并无后代,他又见扁鹊为人善良诚恳,又虚心好学,就把自己的一些医药知识和医疗技术传授给他。

一天,长桑君对扁鹊说:"由于我多年行医游走四方,积累了许多治病救命的秘方,我又没有亲人可以传授,而你与我的关系胜似亲人,我就把这些秘方传授给你,但你千万不能泄露给别人。"扁鹊答应了,于是长桑君就把这些秘方传授给了他。接着长桑君又拿出一包药交给扁鹊:"你用草叶上的露水送服此药,要连着服三十天就能够练成一双慧眼,可以看到平常人看不到的东西。"交代完毕,便与扁鹊告别,飘然远去了。

据传说,按照长桑君的方法,服下了那包药之后,扁鹊能隔着墙看到对面的人。在他给病人看病的时候,能看到病人身体内部器官的病变,经过分析就可判定所生何病,十分准确,从不失误,再对症下药,就达到药到病除的效果。

Sees Through the Crux

Bian Que was a renowned doctor in the Warring States(476 B.C.−221 B.

C.). He had high medical skills and saved many dying people. There were many stories about him in history books and folk tales. But he was not a doctor when he was young. He first worked as a servant in an inn, where he might contact with various people of different trades and occupations. Later, he met a folk called Chang Sang, who had excellent medical skills and often put up for the night in the inn where Bian Que workd, so Bian Que frequently asked for advice from him.

At that time, there was a custom to hand down skills from father to son, of course, including the medical skills. However, Chang Sang was all alone and had no offsprings. He imparted some of his medical skills and techniques to Ban Que, because Bian Que was such a lovely guy, kind, sincere and open-minded.

One day, Chang Sang said to Bian Que, "Since I have been practicing medicine for many years, I've accumulated a lot of secret recipes for life-saving. I don't have any family members to pass on, but our relation is more than relatives. I will give these secret recipes to you, but you cannot reveal to others." So Chang Sang handed down these secret recipes to Bian Que, who had made a promise. Then Chang Sang gave a package of medicines to Bian Que and said, "Taking the medicine with dew on the grass for 30 days, and you are able to see what common people can't see." He bid farewell to Bian Que and went away.

According to the legend, after taking the package of medicine for 30 days, Bian Que was able to see the people through the wall. When he interviewed with a patient, he could see the pathological changes of the internal organs of the patient. So he could find out how the disease came on, and then prescribed the right medicine to cure the disease. His analysis and judgments were very accurate, and never failed.

妙手回春

妙手回春是一个中国成语,比喻医生能够治愈垂死的病人。这是在《荡寇志》第 114 章中说:"根据云先生的说法,刘小姐的病很可能是严重的。恐小生前去,亦属无益……天彪、希真齐声道:'全仗先生妙手回春'。"《官场现形记》第二十回:"什么'妙手回睿',什么'是乃仁术',匾上的字句,一时也记不清楚。"

春秋时期齐国神医扁鹊经过虢国听说虢太子猝死,就问中庶子太子的症状,认为虢太子只是假死可以救活。就叫弟子子阳磨好针,在太子的穴位上扎了几针,太子就苏醒过来,再经汤药调解,20 天后就完全康复,扁鹊赢得"妙手回春"的称号。

Bring a Patient Back to Health

"Bring a patient back to health" is a Chinese idiom. It is a metaphor to describe that a doctor is able to cure a dying patient. Chapter 114 of *Record of Bandits* has this description, "According to Mr. Yun, Miss Liu's illness is likely to be serious. I'm afraid that 'it would make no difference if I go... Tian Biao and Xi Zhen said in chorus that it all depends on your ability of "bringing a patient back to health.'" Chapter 20 of the novel *Exposure of the Official World* also has this saying, "Bringing a patient back to health is a high medical ethic, or something like that. I don't remember clearly the words on the plaque."

During the Spring and Autumn period (770 B.C.–221 B.C.), when Bian Que was passing by the state of Guo, he heard about the sudden death of the prince of the state. After asking the prince's officials about the symptoms of the prince, he analyzed that the prince did not really die and could be saved. So he called his disciple Zi Yang to grind the needles. He performed acupuncture on the prince, and then the prince came to life. After taking medicine for 20 days, the prince recovered completely. Bian Que had won the title of "bringing the dead back to health".

天人相应

"天人相应",从严格意义上说,与"天人合一"论是有区别的。"天人合一"是比较强烈的天命观,天帝意志可以随时体现在社会人事上;"天人相应"或"人与天地相参"则是人以适应自然界规律为主的一种自然天道观。

《吕氏春秋·有始》中说:"天地万物,一人之身也,此之谓大同。"又说:"人与天地也同……故人治身与天下者,必法天地也。"(《情欲》)《荀子》也说:"故善言古者,必有节于今;善言天者,必有征于人。"(《性恶》)《大戴礼记》说:"民与天地相参。"在对天命观的否定过程中,形成了似为折中,实为本质性转变的"天人相应"论。这种"天人相应"、"人与天地相参"的观念,是一种认识论的方法论:即借助于对自然界天地阴阳五行的规律认识来解释和指导人事。同样地,也用来认识人体自身和疾病及治疗。中医理论之所以形成,即由于此方法论的指导;中医理论之所以谓为自然哲学理论,原因也在于此。取类比象,理论根据亦在此。天地大宇宙,人身小宇宙,中医理论在此找到自然生态与人体内环境的统一规律。

Correspondence Between Human and the Nature

The "correspondence between human and the nature", strictly speaking, is not the same as the "syncretism of human and heaven". The latter is a heavenly-destiny view that the will of the heavenly gods can be manifested in society and humanity, at any time. The former is a type of natural view that people should adapt themselves to natural rules.

Described as in Mister Lv's (292 B.C. – 235 B.C.) *Spring and Autumn* bedridden.

When his friend, Yue Guang, knew about that, he remembered that there was a bow hanging on the wall. The snake might be the shadow of the bow reflected in the wine cup. So he invited the guest to his house again. When his friend lifted the cup and saw a snake swimming in the cup, he was extremely amazing. Then Yue Guang told him it was the shadow of the bow on the wall. Then the pressure, like a heavy stone in his heart, was released and his illness was healed.

This story tells us a truth that many diseases are caused by people's suspicion and fear, which can be eliminated by using the "reflection" method.

Annals—Having Start records, "All the things between heaven and earth are just like the human body. This is called the major unity. " It also records in *Lust*, "The human is also a unity of heaven and earth… So people must lead their lives and deal with their affairs under the rule of heaven and earth." Xunzi(313 B.C.-238 B.C.) in *Evil Nature* states, "Those who like citing history must be ruled by the present. Those who like talking about the heaven surely have other people to confirm their evidence." *Dadai Rites* records, "People take heaven and earth as a mirror."In the course of denying the heavenly-destiny view, the theory of correspondence between human and the nature was established in an apparently compromising way, but it signifies a qualitative change in reality. The understanding of a correspondence between human and the nature created an epistemological methodology that recognized the natural rules of *yin-yang* and the five elements—as used to explain and guide human affairs. At the same time, they were used to recognize the human body, its diseases and explain treatment. The formation of Chinese medical theory was thus under the guidance of this methodology and it also explains why Chinese medical theory pertains to natural philosophy. Both the analogical and theoretical foundations of Chinese medicine were formed in this fashion. Heaven and earth are a big universe, while the human body is a small one. Hence, Chinese medicine arrived at the law of unity which existed between the nature and the human body.

悬壶济世

汉代的某年夏天,河南一带闹瘟疫,死了许多人,无法医治。有一天,一个神奇的老人来到这里,他在一条巷子里开了一个小小中药店,门前挂了一个药葫芦,里面盛了药丸,专治这种瘟疫。这位"壶翁"身怀绝技,乐善好施,凡是有人来求医,老人就从药葫芦里摸出一粒药丸,让患者用温开水冲服。就这样,喝了这位"壶翁"药的人,一个一个都好了起来。时有汝南(今河南省平舆县)人费长房,见此老翁在人散后便跳入壶中,他觉得非常奇怪,于是就带了酒菜前去拜访,老翁便邀他同入壶中。费长房从此随其学道,"壶翁"尽授其"悬壶济世"之术。

Xuan Hu Ji Shi (To Practise Medicine to Save People)

In the Han Dynasty (206 B.C.–220 B.C.), there was a plague one summer in Henan. Many people died of the disease. One day, a magical old man came here and opened a small drugstore in an alley. A bottle gourd filled with pills was hung in front of the door. People called him the "Bottle Man". He had unique skills and was kind and generous to everyone. When a patient came up to see him, he took out a pill from the gourd and told him to take it with warm water. All the patients were saved after taking the medicine. There was a man named Fei Changfang, who was born in Runan (Now Pinyu County, Henan Province). He felt strange that the old man jumped into the gourd after people went away. Therefore, Fei came to visit him with food and wine. The old man invited him to go into the gourd. Since then, Fei Changfang became a student of the old man, who taught him the skills to practice medicine to save people.

防微杜渐

《后汉书·丁鸿列传》记载了一则故事:东汉和帝即位时仅十四岁,由于他年幼无能,便由窦太后执政,部分大权实际上落入窦太后的兄弟窦宪等人手中。他们为所欲为,密谋篡权。司徒丁鸿见到这种情况,便上书和帝,建议趁窦氏兄弟权势尚不大时,早加制止,以防后患。

在医学上,防微杜渐体现了预防为主的原则。中医十分重视早期诊治疾病。《内经》说:"善治者治皮毛,其次治肌肤,其次治筋脉,其次治六腑,其次治五脏。"任何疾病都有一个由浅入深的发展过程,高明的医生应该趁疾病轻浅的时候治疗,若疾病已到深重,会变得比较棘手。因此,中医把一个医生是否能对疾病作出早期诊断和治疗当作判断这个医生医技是否高明的标准。

这个成语故事启示我们:隐患要及时清除,以免酿生更大祸端;疾病应及早治疗,以免给机体带来更大的危害。

Be Precautious Before Hand

There was a story in the *Book of Late Han · Biography of Ding Hong* saying, the Eastern Han emperor ascended the throne when he was 14, but because of his young age and incompetence, the government was controlled by the dowager Dou. Actually most power was passed to Dou Xian, brother of dowager Dou. They did what they wanted and even schemed to do away the emperor. Minister Situ Dinghong submitted a written statement to the emperor, suggesting that Dou Xian should be restrained in case of possible future troubles.

In medicine, the idea means the principle of "prevention first". Traditional

Chinese medicine attaches great importance to early diagnosis and treatment. The *Internal Classic* said, "A good doctor first treats the fur, then the skin, muscle, vessel, and finally the six hollow organs and five internal organs." Any disease has a process from mild to severe. A good doctor should give timely treatment while the disease is not serious at the beginning, for the treatment will become more difficult when it becomes severe. Therefore, in traditional Chinese medicine, whether a doctor can make early diagnosis and treatment is regarded as the criterion of his medical skills.

This idiom tells us that the potential dangers should be eliminated in time to avoid the worse situation and the disease should be treated early before it does harm to the body.

贵人难医

　　东汉年间,宫廷御医郭玉的医术高超,经常受到皇帝的嘉奖。郭玉虽身为御医,但见贫苦百姓前来求治,他从不拒绝,而且疗效极好。但令人不解的是,当他为宫中的达官贵人治病时效果反而欠佳。皇帝感到奇怪,便想出一招:令宫中的贵人穿着破旧的衣服,请郭玉来治病,竟然一治而愈。皇帝很不高兴,召郭玉入宫,问其原因。郭玉答道:"行医之道必须精神集中,意念专一,治疗疾病方能得心应手。而给达官贵人治病先有四难:一是不尊重医生的意见,总自以为是。二是生活不规律、不检点。三是体质弱,难于用药。四是好逸恶劳。本来有此四难,就已经难于医治,又加上这些权贵之人对待医生的态度常常是盛气凌人,令人见面便生恐怖之心,所以更是难上加难。就针刺之法而言,本在于心神专注,针刺之深浅仅在于毫微之间。而为贵人治病,常令人心中惶恐不安,手法失度,所以贵人之病难医也。"皇帝听后,不断点头称是,后又责令宫中贵人一一改掉看病陋习。从此,"贵人难医"一说便流传开来。

A Man Is Too Noble To Cure

　　During the Eastern Han Dynasty (25 – 220), Guo Yu, an imperial physician, was often praised by the emperor due to his superb medical skills. Although Guo Yu was an imperial doctor, he never refused to treat the poor, and the effect was excellent. But what puzzled the people was that he was not so successful when he treated the high officials and noble men. The emperor wondered and came up with a small trick. He let the noblemen in the court wear worn-out clothes and asked Guo to see them. However, Guo Yu cured their diseases. The emperor was annoyed and summoned Guo into the palace, asking the whys and wherefores. Guo replied, "The mind of the doctor must be focused when treating diseases. There are four difficulties to treat officials. One is that they do not respect the doctor's opinions. The second is their irregular and undisciplined life. Third, it is difficult to use the medicine because of their weak body. The fourth is that they all indulge in an ease and leisure life rather than physical work. It is difficult to treat those noble men because of the four difficulties, apart from their domineering attitude to their doctors, which made the treatment even more difficult. As far as acupuncture is concerned, it is very important to focus the mind, for a slightest miss is as good as a mile. When treating a noble man, the doctor often feels nervous and the hand is not so accurate in using the needles. So the disease of your distinguished people is difficult to cure." After hearing that, the emperor kept nodding his head and said yes, and then ordered the noblemen in the court to improve their bad habits. From then on, the words "A Man is Too Noble to Cure" spread out.

对症下药

华佗是东汉名医。一次,府吏倪寻和李延两人都患头痛发热,一同去请华佗诊治。华佗经过仔细地望色、诊脉,开出两个不同的处方,交给病人取药回家煎服。两位病人一看处方,给倪寻开的是泻药,而给李延开的是解表发散药。他们想:我俩患的是同一症状,为什么开的药方却不同呢,是不是华佗弄错了? 于是,他们向华佗请教。华佗解释道:倪寻的病是由于饮食过多引起的,病在内部,应当服泻药,将积滞泻去,病就会好;李延的病是受凉感冒引起的,病在外部,应当吃解表药,风寒之邪随汗而去,头痛也就好了。两人听了十分信服。便回家将药熬好服下,果然很快都痊愈了。

中医强调辨证治疗,病症虽一,但引起疾病的原因不同,治疗方法也不一样。后来,人们常用"对症下药"这个成语比喻针对不同情况,采取不同方法处理问题。

Suit the Medicine to the Illness

Hua Tuo was a famous doctor in the Eastern Han Dynasty(25–220). One day, his two inferiors, Ni Xun and Li Yan, both suffered from headache and fever. They went to Hua Tuo for help. Hua carefully inspected and diagnosed them and then prescribed medicinal herbs—two different prescriptions. He gave the medicine to them for home decoction. When the two inferiors got the prescriptions, they both wondered why different treatments were used for the same symptom. Did Hua Tuo make any mistake? So, they went back to see Hua. Hua explained that the differences were due to the different origins of their sickness. Ni's disease was caused by eating too much and his disease was in interior, so he should take laxatives immediately. Li Yan's illness was caused by an exterior cold. He should be given a prescription to relieve exterior syndrome. What Hua said was very convincing and they took the herbs. Sure enough they were cured.

Chinese medicine emphasizes on syndrome differentiation treatment although the symptoms of the disease were the same, but the origins were different. So the treatments should be different, too. Later, people often use the idiom "suit the medicine to the illness" for different situations to take proper steps.

刮骨疗毒

有一次,关羽在战斗中右臂被敌人射中一箭。箭头有毒,毒已入骨,又青又肿,不能动弹。名医华佗听说关羽箭伤不愈,表示能为他割开皮肉,刮骨去毒。手术进行中,华佗刮骨的声音悉悉刺耳,周围的人心惊胆战,掩面失色,而关羽却依然饮酒弈棋,若无其事。等到华佗刮尽骨上的毒,敷上药,缝上线,手术告成,关羽便大笑而起,高兴地说:"先生真是神医。看,我的手臂已经屈伸自如,毫无痛楚了。"华佗也说:"我一生行医,没有见过像您那样沉着坚强的人,真是大丈夫!""刮骨疗毒"后来用作形容意志坚强。

Scrape Poison off the Bone

In a battle, General Guan Yu's right arm was hurt by a poisonous arrow. The toxin had intruded into the bone marrow, and the skin on the spot appeared black and swollen, so his arm was unable to move. Hua Tuo, on hearing Guanyu's injury, proposed to treat the wound. During the operation, the piercing sound from Hua Tuo's scraping bone alarmed all the surrounding soldiers. Nevertheless, Guan Yu was still enjoying drinking and playing chess as if nothing had happened. When Hua Tuo finished scraping the poison off the bone, sewed up and applied medicine to the wound, Guan Yu stood up and said smilingly, "What a good doctor Hua Tuo is! Look, I can move my arm freely and do not feel the pain." Hua Tuo replied, "I've been practicing surgery all my life and have never seen anyone who has such a strong will. You are really a great man!" Since then, the idiom "scrape poison off the bone" is used to describe a man who has a strong will.

杏林春暖

三国时候,吴国侯官中有一位叫董奉的人,是一位医术很高明的医生,传说有"仙术"。他居山不种田,为人治病亦不取钱。重病愈者使栽杏五株,轻者一株。如此数年,得十万余株,蔚然成林。乃使山中百禽群兽游戏其下,后杏子大熟,于林中作一草仓,示时人曰:"欲买杏不须报奉(不用告诉董奉本人),但将一器(容器)谷置仓中,即自往取一器杏去。"常有人置谷来少而取杏去多者,林中群虎出吼逐之,大怖,急走路傍,倾复,至家量杏,一如谷多少。或有人偷杏者,虎逐之,到家啮至死。家人知其偷杏,乃送还奉,叩头谢过,乃却使活。奉每年货杏得谷,旋以账救贫乏,供给行旅不逮者(旅客断了盘费的),岁二万余人。后来董奉"仙去"了。

为了感激董奉的德行,有人写了"杏林春暖"的条幅挂在他家门口。从此,许多中药店都挂上了"杏林春暖"的匾额,"杏林"也逐渐成了中医药行业的代名词。

Xing Lin Chun Nuan

During the Three Kingdoms period(220-280), there was an officer in Wu called Dong Feng. According to the folklore, he was a competent physician and had special skills. He lived in the mountains and did no farm. He cured patients for free. Instead, he asked the patients to plant apricot trees. The severe case was required to plant 5 Xing (apricot) trees while those with milder symptoms one merely. A few years later, the patients who were cured by Dong Feng had planted more than 100,000 apricot trees, which gradually grew into a forest. All the wild animals enjoyed themselves in the forest. When the apricots ripened,

Dong Feng built a storehouse in the forest. He told the local people that if anyone wanted to buy the apricots, he just needed to prepare the same amount of rice to exchange for it and it was not necessary to inform him. However, some people had taken the apricots without putting the equivalent rice back. Thus, the tigers drove these people out of the forest. Those people felt scared and hurried to find a shortcut to come back home. When they got home to weight the apricots, they found that the apricots were as many as the rice. A man stole the apricots and the tiger chased after him. When he came home and ate the apricots, he died. His parents learned the case, sent rice to the storehouse and bent their knees before Dong Feng. Then the dead man came back to life again. Dong used the apricots to exchange rice to help about 20,000 hungry people in a year. Years after, Dong Feng passed away.

To honor Dong's virtues, people sent a scroll "Xing Lin Chun Nuan" (meaning "Spring has come back to the apricot forest") and hung it above his door. Since then, many TCM drugstores hung the plaque "Xing Lin Chun Nuan". So the word "Xing Lin" gradually became the symbol of the Chinese medicine industry.

以毒攻毒

在我国医学历史上,很早就有"免疫"的思想,这就是"以毒攻毒"的治病方法。我国最古老的医学著作《黄帝内经》中提到,治病要用"毒药",药没有"毒"性就治不了病。然而,有趣的是,最早把这种免疫思想付诸于实践,并最早从事免疫学研究的先驱,竟是醉心于炼丹的道教徒葛洪。

葛洪,字稚川,别号朴子。他从小就喜欢读医书和炼丹书,长大后,更在热衷于炼丹术的同时,潜心研究医术,并成了东晋有名的医学家,老百姓有什么急病重病,常找他来医治。

一天,有位40多岁老农急冲冲地来到葛洪的家,焦急地对他说:"我的独生儿子被疯狗咬伤了,请您给想个办法,救他一命。"葛洪听了这话,也很焦急。因为他知道,人若是被疯狗咬伤,会非常痛苦,受不得半点刺激,哪怕是受到一点光,听到一点声音,都能引起抽搐,烦躁,尤其是怕水。听到水,谈到水,见到水,都会立刻咽喉痉挛,发病几小时内便可迅速死亡。葛洪在脑子里搜索着各种各样的药方,但很遗憾没有一个药方能治这种病。忽然,他有了主意:古人不是提倡用"以毒攻毒"的疗法治病吗,为什么不能用疯狗身上的毒物来治这种病呢? 想到这儿,他便对老农说:"现在也没别的什么好办法。不过,我想用疯狗的脑髓涂在你儿子的伤口上,或许能让他脱离危险。"老农回到家后,如法行事。没曾想,还真管用,病人竟没发病。自那以后,葛洪又用这种方法给许多被疯狗咬伤的人治过病,效果挺不错。

近代医学科学证明,在人被狂犬咬伤后,狂犬病毒便通过伤口浸入了人体。由于它与神经组织有特殊的亲和力,所以导致狂犬病的发作。狂犬的脑髓和唾液中,均有大量的狂犬病毒存在。法国著名的生物学家巴斯德便是从狂犬的脑组织中分离出狂犬病毒,并把它加以培养,制成病毒疫苗,来预防和医治狂犬病毒的。很显然,巴斯德所用的原理同葛洪使用的方法基本相似,只不过比葛洪更科学些,但从时间上来看,巴斯德的发明晚于葛洪 1 000 多年。

Fight Poison with Poison

In the history of Chinese medicine, the idea of "immune" appeared long long ago, and that was the method of fighting poison with poison. The oldest medical works in China *The Yellow Emperor's Internal Classic* mentioned that poison can be used in the treatment of diseases, and some diseases can not be cured without poison. However, it was interesting that, the earliest practice of the immune system and the earliest pioneer for immunology was a Taoist called Ge Hong, who was intoxicated in alchemy.

Ge Hong, styled Zhichuan, was also known as Puzi. He preferred to reading medical and alchemy books since childhood. When he grew up, he became more interested in the art of alchemy. At the same time he studied medicine and became a famous medical scientist in the eastern Jin dynasty(317 -420). People who had acute and severe diseases often came to him for help.

One day, an old farmer rushed to Ge Hong's house, saying anxiously that "My only child was bitten by a mad dog. Please save him!" On hearing that, Ge Hong was very anxious, too. He knew that a person, bitten by a mad dog, would be very painful and could not suffer any slightest stimulation, even a little light or a low sound could cause him to convulse, along with irritability and especial fear of water. Hearing the word "water", talking about "water" or seeing water would immediately cause his throat spasm. The patient would die within a few hours. Ge Hong searched all sorts of prescriptions in his brain, but unfortunately no prescription could cure the disease. Suddenly, he had an idea that the ancients advocated to fight poison with poison, which is a therapy to treat some diseases. Why not using the poison from the mad dog to fight this disease?

Then he said to the farmer, "There is no way to do now, but I want to use the mad dog's brains on your son's wound, which perhaps would get him out of danger." The farmer did so after returning home. It was surprising that this method worked and the patient was finally cured. Since then, Ge Hong used this method to cure many people who got bitten by mad dogs and it worked quite well.

It has been shown that after the man is bitten by a rabid dog, the rabies virus will immerse into the human body through the wound. Rabies virus and nerve tissue have special affinity, so it causes the outbreak of rabies. There is a large number of rabies virus in the brains and saliva of the rabid dog. The famous French biologist, Pasteur, isolated rabies from the brains of a rabid dog and cultivated it to make a viral vaccine to prevent and treat rabies. It is obvious that Pasteur's method was more scientific, though similar to that of Ge Hong's. But Pasteur's invention was more than 1,000 years later than Ge Hong's.

杯弓蛇影

《晋书·乐广传》记载,一天,乐广宴请宾客,大厅中觥筹交错,异常热闹。大家猜拳行令,饮酒作乐。一位客人正举杯痛饮,无意中瞥见杯中似有一游动的小蛇,但碍于众多客人的情面,他硬着头皮把酒喝下。从此以后,他忧心忡忡,老是觉得有蛇在腹中蠢蠢欲动,恶心欲吐,最后竟卧床不起。

乐广得知他的病情后,思前想后,终于记起他家墙上挂有一张弯弓,他猜测这位朋友所说的蛇一定是倒映在酒杯中的弓影,于是,他再次把客人请到家中,邀朋友举杯,那个朋友刚举起杯子,墙上弯弓的影子又映入杯中,宛如一条游动的小蛇,他惊得目瞪口呆,乐广这才把事情的原委告诉了他,病人疑窦顿开,压在心上的石头被搬掉,病也随之而愈。

这个故事意在告诉人们这么一个道理,说明人在很多时候都是疑神疑鬼的,而由这种怀疑和恐惧所引起的疾病,可以用"深思"的方法来解除其紧张恐惧的心理状态,从而使疾病消除,恢复健康。

Mistake the Shadow of a Bow in One's Cup As a Snake

According to the record in *Book of Jin · A Biography of Yue Guang*, one day, Yue Guang invited many guests to his house. The guests were drinking happily and playing the finger guessing game. The house was filled with joy. A guest suddenly caught a glimpse of a small snake moving in his wine cup. However, in order not to disturb other guests, he forced himself to drink up the wine. After that, he was always anxious that there was a small snake swimming in his stomach, which made him nauseous to vomit. Finally, he was completely bedridden.

When his friend, Yue Guang, knew about that, he remembered that there was a bow hanging on the wall. The snake might be the shadow of the bow reflected in the wine cup. So he invited the guest to his house again. When his friend lifted the cup and saw a snake swimming in the cup, he was extremely amazing. Then Yue Guang told him it was the shadow of the bow on the wall. Then the pressure, like a heavy stone in his heart, was released and his illness was healed.

This story tells us a truth that many diseases are caused by people's suspicion and fear, which can be eliminated by using the "reflection" method.

骗子卖药

柳宗元患病,请来一位名医诊治。医生说:"你的脾脏肿大,吃些上等的茯苓就会好的!"柳宗元派人去药店买来茯苓,煎成汤药喝了下去。哪知道病情不但没有减轻,反而更加重了。

柳宗元以为是医生误用了药,就把医生叫来,责问他是怎么回事。医生不信自己误用了药,把药罐里的药渣倒出来验看。原来不是茯苓,而是经过加工染色的老山芋干。医生叹了口气说:"卖药的是个骗子,吃药的又不识货,光靠医生是治不好病的!"

A Swindler Sold Herbs

Once Liu Zongyuan (773-819), a famous writer, was ill. He called on a famous doctor for diagnosis and treatment. The doctor said, "Your spleen is swollen. You will get well by taking some good quality *fuling* (poria cocos)." Liu Zongyuan sent someone to buy *fuling* from a drug store, boiled it and drank the decoction. However, his illness was not relieved, but turned worse instead.

Thinking that the doctor had prescribed the wrong medicine, he called on and reproved him again, asking what the matter was. The doctor didn't believe this. He poured out the dregs of the decoction from the pot and examined them. To his surprise, they were not *fuling*, but just dried sweet potatoes, dyed and processed. The doctor sighed and said, "Illness cannot be cured by the doctor alone if the herb seller is a swindler and the medicine taker does not know head or tail of it."

怡悦疗法

相传金元时期名医张子和善治疑难杂症。一个名叫项关令的人来求诊,说他夫人得了一种怪病,只知道腹中饥饿,却不想进食饭菜,整天大喊大叫,喜怒无常,吃了许多药,都无济于事。张子和听后,认为此病服药难以奏效,就告诉病人家属,得找来两名妇女,令装扮成演戏的丑角,故作姿态,扭扭捏捏地做出许多滑稽动作。如此一来,果然令病人心情怡悦。接着,张子和又叫病人家属请来两位食欲旺盛的妇女,在病人面前狼吞虎咽地吃东西。病人看着看着,也不知不觉地跟着吃起来。就这样,张子和利用怡悦引导之法,使该妇人心情逐渐平和稳定,最终不药而愈。

Pleasure Therapy

As legend has it that during the Jin and Yuan Dynasties(1115 – 1368), a famous doctor named Zhang Zihe(1156 – 1228) was good at treating difficult diseases. A man named Xiang Guanling came to see him and said that his wife was suffering from a strange disease. She felt hungry but did not want to eat any food. She shouted all day long and snarled angrily. His wife ate a lot of medicine with no effect at all. After hearing this, Zhang Zihe decided to seek for two women to dress up as clowns in a drama. This really made the patient happy. Then Zhang and the family invited two women with strong appetites to devour food in front of the sick lady. The patient watched and began to eat unconsciously. In this way, the woman became calm and stable gradually. She was cured without taking any medicine.

激怒疗法

传说战国时代的齐闵王患了忧郁证,请宋国名医文挚来诊治。文挚详细诊断后,告诉太子说:"齐王的病只有用激怒的方法来治疗才能治好。只是我激怒了齐王,他肯定要把我杀死的。"太子听说父王有救,一再恳求道:"只要能治好父王的病,我和母后一定会保证你的生命安全。"文挚推辞不过,只得应允。当即与齐王约好看病的时间。结果文挚第一次没有来,又约第二次;第二次也没来又约第三次;第三次同样失约。

齐闵王见文挚丝毫不尊重自己,总请不到,连续三次失约,非常恼怒,痛骂文挚不止。过了几天,文挚突然来了,连礼也不见,鞋也不脱,就踩上齐王的床铺问疾看病,并且用粗话野话激怒齐王。齐王实在忍耐不住了,便起身大骂文挚,一怒一骂,郁闷一泄,齐王的忧郁症也就好了。只可惜,太子和他的母后并没有保住文挚的性命,齐闵王还是因文挚不敬,愤怒地把他给杀了。

文挚根据中医情志治病的"怒胜思"的原则,采用激怒病人的治疗手段,却治好了齐王的忧郁证,给传统医学医案史上留下了一个心理疗法的典型范例。

Anger Therapy

As legend has it that Emperor Qimin(? -284 B.C.) of the Warring States period suffered from depression syndrome. He invited a famous doctor of Song (1114 B.C.-286 B.C) named Wen Zhi to treat him. After a detailed diagnosis, Wen Zhi told the prince,"The king's illness can only be cured by a method of provocation. But once I provoke him, he will surely kill me." Knowing that this could save his father's life, the prince begged again and again, "As long as you can save my father, my mother and I will guarantee your safety." Wen agreed and made an appointment with the king. Wen Zhi did not appear at the appointment for the first and second time, the third time either.

Emperor Qi Min saw that Wen Zhi did not respect him and had broken his promise three times in succession, he was very angry and scolded Wen Zhi more than once. A few days passed, Wen came to see the emperor unexpectedly. He did not take off his shoes and stepped on the king's bed and irritated him by using rude words. The king could not bear him any longer. He stood up impatiently and swore loudly at Wen, which gave vent to his depression. In this way Emperor Qi Min was recovered from his illness. Unfortunately, the prince and his mother could not save the life of Wen Zhi. The king killed him for disrespecting.

According to the TCM principle "Anger is better than thought" in treating emotional diseases, Wen Zhi cured the depression of Emperor Qi by irritating him, which was a typical example of psychotherapy in the history of traditional medicine.

逗笑疗法

据说清代有位巡按大人患了精神抑郁症,终日愁眉不展,病情日趋严重。其下属及家人到处为他寻医问药,始终不见疗效。某日,有位幕僚推荐一位乡野老郎中来帮他看病。老郎中望闻问切一番后,平静地对这位闷闷不乐的巡按大人说:"你得的是月经不调啊,别着急,用点乌鸡白凤丸,再加调养调养就会好的。"巡按听了捧腹大笑,心里嘀咕这老郎中真是个糊涂医生啊,连男女都分不清。此后,巡按经常拿老郎中说事,说这郎中真是荒唐,让男人服用乌鸡白凤丸调经。每每想起此事,他就不禁暗自发笑。久而久之,他的抑郁证居然不药而愈了。这时候,老郎中回来了,并对巡按说:"大人,因为你这个病啊,是郁则气结所致。并没有什么良药,只能靠心情愉快才有可能治好。我说你患了月经不调,只是想让大人经常开怀大笑,直至不药而愈啊。"巡按大人这才恍然大悟,连忙道谢。称赞老郎中出手不凡,果然医术高明。

Fun Therapy

It is said that in the Qing Dynasty(1636-1912) there was a government official, who suffered from mental depression and was worried all day long. His family and subordinates went around to seek medical treatment for him, but reached no curative effect. One day, a staff recommended an old rural doctor to see him. The old man checked him carefully and said to the worried official calmly, "You suffered from the irregular menstruation. Don't worry and take some Wuji Baifeng pills, and you will be fine." The official was convulsed with laughter for such a confused practitioner that he can't tell a man from a woman.

Since then, the practitioner was mentioned again and again for his absurd prescription of using Wuji Baifeng pills to regulate a man's menstruation. Whenever he thought about it, he could not help laughing in his heart. In the end, his depression was cured without taking any medicine at all. At this time the old man returned and said to him, "Because your illness is the combination of grief and anger, there is no good medicine for it. And it can only be cured by being in a good mood." The official suddenly saw the light and praised highly for the fine skill of the old doctor.

羞耻疗法

羞耻是人的本能,尤其是古代女子。传说有一民间年轻女子,因打哈欠,两手上举后,再也不能放下来。家人到处求医问诊,中药针灸治疗旬月,竟然皆无效果。后请来名医俞用右视病。这俞用右医师便利用了女子害羞的心理特点,扬言要为她作针灸治疗,并慢慢打开了针灸包。甚至伸出双手做出要给女子解裤带脱裤子的动作来。这女子被这突如其来的手势动作给吓坏了。出于害羞的本能,她不自觉地急忙用双手提拉自己的衣裤并护着下身私处。如此,双手顺势自然下垂而复原了。这种"声东击西"的情志疗法,果然收到了意想不到的效果。

Shame Therapy

Shame is a human instinct, especially for ancient Chinese women. As legend has it that a young woman's hands could no longer be put down after yawning with hands raised. Her family sought various kinds of medical treatment for her for ten days, with no effect. At last, a very famous doctor named Yu Yongyou was invited to see her. Doctor Yu understood that shyness is a female instinct. He pretended to make acupuncture treatment for her, opened the acupuncture package slowly, and then stretched out his hands to unfasten her pants belt, pretending to take off the woman's pants. The woman was frightened by the sudden gesture. Out of the instinct of shyness, she hurried to pull her clothes and trousers with both hands, trying to protect her private parts. In this way, her hands naturally drooped down. This emotional therapy of "making a feint to the east and attacking the west" has really received unexpected results.

参考文献

［1］李照国,朱忠宝.中医英语翻译技巧训练［M］.上海：上海中医药大学出版社,2002.

［2］李照国.译海心语［M］.上海：上海中医药大学出版社,2006.

［3］李照国.中医基本名词术语英译标准化研究：理论研究、实践总结、方法探索［M］.上海：上海科学技术出版社,2008.

［4］史志南,奚亚夫.汉英对照中国古代故事精选集［M］.上海：复旦大学出版社,1997.

［5］王方路.唐诗三百首白话英语双译探索［M］.上海：复旦大学出版社,2010.

［6］许渊冲.汉英对照唐宋词一百首［M］.北京：中国对外翻译出版公司,1991.

［7］杨立义.中国成语故事一百篇［M］.北京：中国对外翻译出版公司,1991.

［8］周仪.中国文化故事［M］.上海：同济大学出版社,2012.